ANGUS CUNNINGHAM

TWICE BEFORE
TWELVE
A JOURNEY THROUGH CHILDHOOD CANCER

Copyright © 2026 by Angus Cunningham

All rights reserved. Apart from fair dealing for the purposes of study, research, criticism or review as permitted under the Copyright Act, no part of this publication may be reproduced, distributed or transmitted in any form or by any means without prior written permission.

The information in this book is not intended to replace professional medical or psychological advice. The content is based upon the author's personal experiences, opinions and qualifications.

All necessary written permissions have been obtained from others to publish their stories. Some names have been changed to protect identities, whereas others have asked that their real names be used.

Cover design by Judith San Nicolas
Typeset in Garamond 9/12pt & Verdana 22pt
Printed and bound in Australia by IngramSpark
Prepared for publication by Dr Juliette Lachemeier @ The Erudite Pen Independent Publishing

A catalogue record for this book is available from the National Library of Australia

Twice Before Twelve: A Journey Through Childhood Cancer – 1st edition
ISBN Paperback 9781764337809
ISBN Ebook 9781764337816

Dedication

To Mum and Dad.

You supported me in ways no parent should ever have to. Without you, I don't know where I would be or what I would do. This story is as much yours as it is mine, and I hope you enjoy it.

Foreword

When we started Rare Cancers Australia (RCA) in 2012 we knew that one of the most vulnerable groups in the cancer community were those families dealing with a childhood cancer. Every child's cancer is rare and that creates many problems. Funding for treatment and research is always difficult to find. Collecting enough patients with the same cancer to test new therapies thoroughly requires international co-operation, and treatment and research only takes place in a few major centers around the world.

But the major challenge is the impact on the child and their family. Excruciating treatments are delivered to patients that are too young to understand what is happening, whilst their parents and family are forced to sit and watch, powerless to intervene and struggling to understand. New treatments that are available are only available at exorbitant cost because our health system is too rigid.

Parents are programmed to protect and nurture their children and yet when their child has cancer, they become a spectator and supporter. They try to guess what their child is thinking and suffering whilst they deal with their frustrations and powerlessness. But no more, as this book provides everyone with an insight not only into Angus's state of mind as he navigated through his cancer journey but as importantly, a look inside the mind of a child undergoing treatment, and it does so with extraordinary clarity and eloquence. It is compulsory reading for anyone living or working with children and cancer.

His story also provides us with an understanding of what we lose when we don't invest enough in the health of our children. Angus is an extraordinary young man who will doubtless make a huge contribution to Australia during the twenty-first century. It is unthinkable that we could have lost him because our government and a pharmaceutical company couldn't agree on a price to treat him. Angus and the Cunningham Family are extraordinary Australians, not only did they allow RCA to raise money for Angus's treatment, but they generated a surplus that helped so many more patients in need.

Parts of this book are raw and confronting but it captures the incredible spirit and optimism that is Angus. We are lucky to have him in both senses of the word and there is no doubt we will be hearing lots more of him in the future, thankfully.

Richard and Kate, Founders, Rare Cancers Australia

CONTENTS

Introduction 1
The First Diagnosis 3
One of Many 7
That Fateful Day 13
Goodbye, Hair 23
The Starlight Room 31
Great White or Bull Shark? 41
More Needles 47
Intermission 53
Life Goes On 61
The Calm Before the Storm 73
The Second Diagnosis 77
Not as Straightforward 87
Managing Anxiety 97
The ICE Cycle 107
Stem Cell Harvest 115
Michael Ennis Visits 121
Radiotherapy 129
A Ray of Hope 139
A Touch of Normality 147
Crack! 155
Isolation Month Begins 167

The Long Haul	175
New Routine	185
Goodbye, Chemo Hello, Stem Cells	193
Worse Before Better	205
Return of the White Blood Cells	217
Surprise!	229
End of Isolation	243
Hitting a Snag	257
Rooster	267
A New Set of Challenges	273
An Odd Year	285
A New Path	293
Photo Gallery	303
Acknowledgements	327

Introduction

Hello, my name is Angus Cunningham and at the time of writing this book, I am twenty years old. This is the story of how I stared down childhood cancer – not once, but twice – and came out the other side forever changed. It tested everything I had, but it also gave me a deeper strength, a sharper perspective and a new appreciation for life I never expected to find.

Cancer first appeared in my life when I was ten years old, and then I relapsed when I was twelve. There was a seven per cent chance of my cancer relapsing after initial treatment, and I fell into that category. It drastically changed the trajectory of my life.

That being said, I am not writing my story to gain any sympathy from anyone because, in a weird way, I am appreciative for everything I have endured. I believe that what happened to me as a child helped me become deeply grateful for every single day I have on this earth. It's not an easy mindset to develop, especially with how challenging life can be at times, but I felt blessed to have learned that perspective early on.

There have been enough tears shed by my family and me, so if there's anything I'd like you take out of my story, I want it to be gratitude and positivity. I live my life by these two guiding principles, and I strongly believe that a positive mindset and attitude can help build resilience, which in this life is something that can take you anywhere. Resilience will be a common theme throughout my story, and I believe that everyone has resilience in them, no matter how dire their situations may seem.

I hope that by reading my story, you feel inspired and understand how important it is to be there for one another, especially when situations become tough. I've been privileged to witness firsthand the incredible strength of a community and the profound impact we can have when we support one another. This is especially true when being there for others, as my mum always told me, 'Being nice goes a long way'.

Oh, and, if you ask anyone who knows me, I like to yap on a lot! But my editor assures me she will rein this in for your sakes.

With that said, let's dive into my story.

The First Diagnosis

My story starts when I was just nine years old. Looking back, I loved my life. I can't remember a time in my childhood when I was ever sad or upset. I come from a loving family: Trish and Steve, my parents, and my three brothers Henry, Noah and Darcy. Yes, that is correct, four boys. Funny enough, our names in order spell HAND: Henry, Angus, Noah and Darcy. Pure coincidence, apparently (nice try, Mum).

Mum and Dad were always busy; at the time Mum was a lawyer and Dad was a physiotherapist, but they still always made time for us. If they couldn't take care of us, my beautiful grandparents Fran and Rodney Cashmere (Mum's parents) and Mary and Barry Cunningham (Dad's parents) or family friends would step in to help. I love both of my grandparents very much. We were always supported growing up, and I feel lucky when I sit here and reflect on my childhood. My best mate when I was younger was my older brother Henry. Growing up, I always looked up to him. We were only three years apart in age and had very similar interests. I wanted to be just like him, mimicking everything he did, whether it was copying his haircuts or even stealing his clothes.

Funnily enough, this innocent idolisation of my older brother was the reason I first discovered the lumps.

For context, Henry had a benign lump on his ribs that he was born with. It was completely fine to leave it there, and he had just grown up with it being there with no issue. But as the younger brother, I remember being jealous of this lump. I know, right? I was jealous of a lump; it's laughable now, but at the time, I thought that lump was the coolest thing in the world. So, you could imagine how excited I was to one day find a set of lumps on my neck the size of golf balls. *I am now just like my older brother*, I remember thinking to myself. I thought it was so cool, and I was so excited; however, my parents didn't feel the same way about these mysterious lumps…

It was around March or April 2013 when the first lumps appeared. Soon after, I found myself sitting in my local GP's office, where a routine check quickly turned serious, prompting the immediate order of blood tests. To our relief, the blood tests were completely fine, and with me being such a fit and healthy kid, we were told that there was little to worry about. We were advised that if any other symptoms occur or the lumps don't go away, then to come back for more investigation.

So, for a little while, I carried on with my life, with my parents monitoring the lumps. At the time, I was playing rugby league and like any kid from Sydney around that age, I dreamed of growing up and playing in the NRL for the Cronulla Sharks. I was also a very passionate skateboarder and would practise from sunup to sundown. My days were filled with rugby league and skateboarding, and I wouldn't stop until I caught the ball just right or nailed the trick. I chased perfection, practising until there were no mistakes left to make. That was just the kind of kid I was: work hard, stay focused and trust that the results would come. This mindset was instilled in me from a young age, and it stuck.

After a few weeks had passed, there was still no regression of the lumps whatsoever. They had, if anything, gotten bigger every day. My mum then took me back to the GP for further testing, as she was always caring for us boys and wanted to make sure that we were okay. That's just the type of person Mum is, always putting everyone above herself, which will be a consistent trait throughout this story.

By early July 2013, I was ten years old, and the ultrasound had been completed. The results were inconclusive, with nothing coming up. The scans only revealed swelling in the lymph nodes on both sides of my neck. Nothing else. By this time, it had been months since I had noticed the lymph nodes in my neck.

I never really stressed about it, either. I don't know if it was just because I was a naive kid or too busy caught up with my life. Who knows? It was probably a mix of both. This set of negative results, plus countless blood tests that came back inconclusive, was enough for my parents and my GP. There was some debate about whether I was going to get a needle biopsy or a lymphadenectomy. The first option, the needle biopsy, is when a practitioner puts a needle directly into the lymph node to take out some fluid, then test what is going on inside them. The second option, the lymphadenectomy, is a surgery where a surgeon cuts open a part of the body to remove a few lymph nodes for dissection. In my case, it was going to be my neck where they would operate. You could imagine as a ten-year-old child that I was not too keen on a needle being shoved into my neck, so option two was the way in which we were going forward.

The surgery was booked for the 29th of July. We were reassured and almost relieved to have, in our eyes, a final date to find out what was going on. We were finally going to receive answers after months of worry from my parents, and this entire mishap was going to come to an end. But little did we know that this was just the start of our journey.

One of Many

The 29th of July came around soon enough, and the surgery was only going to be a short day procedure. I would be home by the afternoon. I was excited to be in the hospital for the first time because I was an energetic, curious kid. To my parent's surprise (and looking back, to my surprise), I'd had no previous hospital visits, not even for any broken bones or anything. So this new hospital experience excited me.

All four of us boys didn't really have any times where we got injured. The only injury we experienced was when my older brother, Henry, split his knee open in Singapore on the final day of our holiday. Dad had been supposed to watch us for an hour, and in that hour, Henry managed to slip over in the pool and need stitches. The only other time that I can think of one of us getting injured was actually, ironically, my fault. I was playing with my two younger brothers Noah and Darcy, and like the talented rugby league player I was, I decided to ankle tap Noah. To cut a short story shorter, he came out second best with a clean break of his collarbone. Mum was also on holiday then, so let's just say Dad is two for two when looking after us boys. Sorry to throw you under the bus, Dad!

The surgery went as well as possible, and I remember thinking about what I would do next. I had to take a few weeks off from playing footy to let the stitches heal, but I was determined to make up for it by playing my best when I returned. I still rocked up to support my teammates from the sideline, as I loved being a part of a team. Little did I know, though, that the last game I played before the surgery was unfortunately going to be my last for the rest of the year.

We were booked into the Sydney Children's Hospital in early August 2013 to get the results of the surgery. Mum and Dad both came with me, which I thought was a little bit odd because one of them was usually working or busy. Thinking back to that day, everything seemed like a massive blur. I remember sitting in the waiting room with my parents. I couldn't tell if my parents were nervous or not, but I certainly wasn't. I didn't feel fazed one bit. After speaking with them later, they were extremely on edge, but the last thing they wanted to do was worry me. I didn't have a care in the world; all that was on my mind was getting back to my sports and school.

We were only waiting for about ten to twenty minutes before a nurse in a full blue gown yelled out my name, meaning it was my time. I remember looking at the nurse who was leading us into the room; she had a giant smile on her face, not one bit of angst or anything that seemed off at all. We were then led into a private consult room, where my surgeon was sitting. She was beaming with joy, clearly pleased to see us. This smile eased my parents' worries and comforted them; nonetheless, something still felt off. All the health professionals had seemed so untroubled, and looking back, it must've been the calm before the storm. As my mum came to later explain to me, 'We were deceived by the belief that a smile meant we were fine. That smile signalled our lives would change forever.'

The surgeon greeted us and we sat down. A conversation had brewed between my parents and the surgeon, but I wasn't involved. As I stated earlier, I was always a curious kid and loved learning, but for whatever reason that day, once I entered the room, I became so distant. I don't know why, but I simply remember everything in that room as a blur, and my heart was pounding at an accelerated pace. My head was hot, and I felt like I was going to be sick. I'm not sure why I felt this way, given that I was completely unaware of the daunting situation unfolding around me, but something felt amiss. The calm demeanour I'd had just moments before was now completely gone.

I started coming to a bit, and I just remembered the sheer look of fear in my parents' eyes. This scary word kept getting thrown around. CANCER. This six-letter word. It didn't seem real. As a kid, I thought cancer was something only older people got. My beautiful grandma, Fran, had beaten breast cancer the year before, so in my mind, it was something that only happened to adults. *Will I still get to go to school? Can I still play footy? Can I still participate in the cross country coming up?* Funnily enough, those were my first thoughts. It really shows just how innocent and unaware I was in the middle of something so serious.

I was diagnosed with Classical Hodgkin Lymphoma, nodular sclerosing type. I had stage 2A, as it was on both sides of my neck. Not long after the surgeon informed us of my diagnosis, we were introduced to a wonderful man by the name of Toby Trahair. Based on what I remember, he appeared from behind the door, kind of like an angel. I don't recall him walking through the door, because at that moment, I was a prisoner in my own mind, my thoughts racing a thousand kilometres per hour. 'Dr Toby Trahair is a paediatric oncologist who specialises in kids' cancer,' we were assured. A complete stranger at the time, Dr Trahair was, but little did we know we were going to get to know him very, very well.

Toby, who insisted we call him by his first name and not Dr Trahair, attempted to reassure us everything would be okay as Mum, Dad and I sat frozen in shock. We couldn't believe it. How could a young, healthy kid get such a catastrophic disease as this? My parents fed me a clean diet and I exercised daily. Isn't this meant to stop you from getting sick? So many questions, with so few answers. Toby then proceeded to explain how this cancer was treatable and that a cure was achievable.

This helped to ease my parents a little bit; however, I was still silent. I didn't know what to say. I was overwhelmed, which was a weird feeling, I'll tell you. Not only that, but I'd never really had any health issues before this, so it was an extremely new concept to me. The conversation ended with Toby's famous line: 'Questions?'

This simple phrase would become the signature finish to every meeting we ever had with him. It was a calming moment, much like Toby himself, a smart, soft-spoken man who always knew how to help us feel at ease. His quiet confidence created an environment where we felt comfortable asking anything, turning what could have been intimidating meetings into relaxed discussions. Each time he uttered that word, it was a gentle invitation to dive deeper, assuring us that our thoughts and concerns were valued.

Before continuing with my story, I want to take a moment to explore some statistics on childhood cancer in Australia. This topic interests me, and as I write this, I'm curious to explore how many children are affected by cancer and the survival rates.

Here are some confronting facts about childhood cancer:
- For every 10 children diagnosed with cancer, 2 don't survive.
- Most children (two-thirds) who actually survive cancer still battle with lifelong health issues as a result of their treatment.
- My cancer, Hodgkin lymphoma, is rare in children, as the most common age is 39 years old.

- Cancer kills more children than any other disease in Australia.[1]

I'm honestly blown away by those statistics. It's crazy to think that just over a thousand kids go through something like this each year. These are quite confronting statistics. Now let's get back to my story as my journey echoes many of these children's.

---

[1] https://www.ccia.org.au/about-childhood-cancer; https://www.canceraustralia.gov.au/cancer-types/childrens-cancer/types-childrens-cancer/hodgkin-lymphoma-hodgkin-disease

That Fateful Day

After leaving the hospital, the walk back to the car was once again a blur. On that fateful day, my memory is understandably very hazy. All I can remember is the sheer shock that all of us were feeling. It was an indescribable feeling. As humans, it's natural and normal to plan for the future, but in an instant, my future was no longer guaranteed. I couldn't even think about a birthday party for next week or a dinner for Friday, let alone long-term future goals. This day was going to drastically change my life, and the everlasting effects will be felt forever by myself and my family.

The next day, as you can imagine, came with such a weird feeling. I remember being at school and having only told my closest friends at the time that something was wrong. My parents opted to keep this semi-private, only really telling our close friends and family at the time. Little did we know, however, the impact this would have on everyone around us and the support our community and the nation would give us. At the time though, we made the decision to keep it confidential.

It was a completely unfamiliar situation for us and for everyone we knew. Even though the Sutherland Shire, about twenty-five kilometres south of the Sydney CBD, is a big area, it has that small-town feeling where everyone seems to know each other. Yet at the time, no one in our circle had ever faced childhood cancer. That made the whole experience feel even more isolating and daunting. We were stepping into the unknown, unsure of what to expect or what might happen.

Even at my young age, I had many questions, with little to no answers. Mum and Dad were trying to shelter me from the harsh realities that come along with cancer treatment. I just wanted to be a normal kid and play with my friends. At first, after that initial diagnosis, it was the worst time, just seeing how it affected everyone I loved. It was honestly torture. I would wake up some nights and have one of my parents next to me in tears; it was terrible, and I wouldn't wish it on my worst enemy. My pillow would be drenched from tears, and I would feel helpless as there was nothing I could do to make them not cry. But it made me determined that I just had to get better. *They don't deserve this pain I am putting them through*, I used to think to myself, *not one bit*.

Even though the surgeries had little recovery time, I felt abnormal and like a bit of an outsider. This wasn't anyone's fault, and it would break my parents' hearts to hear me say that I felt this way, but it's just how I felt. When you're ten years old and in Year 4, you want to go out and be active and play with your friends. That was just the normal thing to do. Nonetheless, I was about to endure chemotherapy treatment, which was going to make not standing out a whole lot harder.

Dr Trahair (Toby) organised a PET scan to see where the cancer had spread to so he could tell us what stage of cancer I had. To those of you who've been unfortunate enough to have had a PET scan, I sympathise with you. It is a full process to have one of these bastards of a scan. Firstly, you have to fast for around six hours before the scan, so you're dying to eat food. They then require you to sit completely still in a chair while the staff intravenously administer a radioactive solution that enhances the quality of the images. You must drink a lot of this yellow liquid to ensure a clear scan. After this checklist, then you are finally ready for the scan. Sound exciting yet? Well, after all this, they need you to remain hot. Yes, that is correct. Not in the looks department, because I'm sure I had that covered with my Justin Bieber haircut, but actually *hot*.

They wrap you in heated blankets, ensuring you remain warm until the scan concludes. I haven't even mentioned the best part yet! You have to sit completely still in a big machine that covers your whole body for around forty minutes while dripping in sweat. I remember feeling so claustrophobic but had to put on a brave face as I could see the fear on Mum and Dad's faces. That's the worst part, seeing the people you love worried and in fear.

Anyway, at the conclusion of the scan, I was once again allowed to eat, so it was hospital sandwiches for me. I can't lie, the ham sandwich wasn't too bad, and I could definitely have eaten a few more of them. Looking at a PET scan is such a daunting process. I will never forget my first glimpse of the nasty cancer cells that had engulfed both sides of my neck. I could feel the dark shadows lurking inside my body. The cancer cells glowed like hidden embers in a field of ash, small but ominous signals of the danger lurking beneath the surface. The scan results were clear: stage 2A Hodgkin lymphoma, which, considering all things, was a good result. Toby's words, *'Cancer is treatable,'* kept replaying in my head like a broken record. This brought some peace to my young mind, though little did we know what lay ahead.

Wednesday 14, August 2013 09:55:25 Trisha Cashmere <t*******cashmere**@gmail.com>wrote:

Subject: Just an update with what is happening with Angus….

To our wonderful friends and family

We just spent 80 minutes speaking to the oncologist (thanks, Debbie, I conference-called in). The side effects of treatment were explained, and we were reassured that the prognosis is excellent. Angus has been staged at IIA.

Chemotherapy will be starting tomorrow. There will be two cycles of four weeks where he will receive one of four drugs on day 8 and day 15. This means he will be in hospital now until Sunday night. Then back for the treatment on Monday, Tuesday and Thursday of next week.

Angus will lose his hair, probably in about two to three weeks. Other than that, it's wait and see. There are a number of short-term side effects that may or may not occur. He will need to take it easy, no contact sport for a while, and no shopping centres. If he is exposed to chickenpox or measles, he needs prophylactic treatment, so if you become aware of anyone with these conditions in our community, please let me know. He will be at school when he feels up to it. He may be a bit grumpy.

This will be the first of what we hope will only be two rounds of treatment.

Our plan is that Steve or I will be with Angus whenever he is in hospital, and the other will be keeping the home going. We are both fortunate to be able to take time off work.

I've just let Sally R know that all those kind offers of meals would now be helpful (she is coordinating this for us).

I may have forgotten someone. My brain is a little frazzled, please let those who would like to know what is happening. You may forward on this email.

Thank you all for the kindness and support. We have been overwhelmed.

Other than that, wish us luck and please look out for my other beautiful boys.

Trisha xx

The orders were in: On the 14th of August, I was to book in a surgery and get a portacath put into the right side of my chest. For the people who don't know what a portacath is, here is the definition: A portacath is a small device typically implanted beneath the skin on the right side of the chest. It's connected to a thin, flexible tube, or catheter, which is inserted into a large vein located above the heart, known as the superior vena cava. It looks like a small bump underneath your skin below your right pec. Portacaths were put in to administer intravenous fluids and blood transfusions, and give me chemotherapy. They remained in place for extended periods of time, so this minimised the need for frequent needles. It was a pretty handy little device, and it wasn't too noticeable; however, they can have their issues, which you'll come to find later on. I found out firsthand.

So, my first lot of treatments in 2013 involved chemotherapy. The day following my portacath implant, I began my treatment. Doctor Toby had instructed that I was to follow a trial at the time known as the GPOH HD 2002. This trial had the best results with as few side effects as possible, but with chemotherapies, the list is still in the hundreds of possible consequences.

At the time, I was classified as a low-risk patient, which meant that if a clear PET scan was visible after the chemotherapies, I would avoid radiation. This is the best possible result, as radiation can be devastating and have severe long-term effects that carry on for the rest of a person's life. Now let me try and name all the drugs that I was given. Don't ask me to explain what they did or what any of the side effects were; I just know that they were was meant to help me. My first exposure to this poisonous cocktail included: Two cycles of OEPA Chemotherapy (vincristine, etoposide, prednisone, doxorubicin), with the first cycle commencing in August and the second cycle in September. The cycle was to be given every twenty-eight days.

Here's a fun fact: I'm not sure which chemotherapy I received during my treatment, but one of them was originally an ingredient in mustard gas! As a history fanatic, I found it fascinating to discover that a treatment I was undergoing had such a dark history as a World War One weapon.

I remember the day I had my first chemotherapy. I was lying down when a group of nurses suddenly entered the room. The nurses appeared prepared for the procedure, clad in purple gowns that concealed their clothing, with eye protection and gloves. The chemo was even covered with grey duct tape; that's right, the bags it came in had to be covered as human skin couldn't come into contact with it. Well, only mine was allowed to.

The first week went as smoothly as it could go. My body was tolerating the cocktail of chemotherapies that I was having. I kept on thinking, *I am not going to lose my hair or get sick.* I was always telling Toby (my oncologist) that I felt fine and well up to participating in sports. It's kind of sad, isn't it? At such a young age, I never truly understood what I was fighting against or even realised that I was in the fight of my life. However, I wouldn't change it for the world, as this allowed me to always be in a positive mindset, which would come to significantly help me. The countdown was on until the hair would fall out. To be honest, losing my hair was my only stress. As I mentioned before, I had the Bieber fringe going on, so the thought of losing that was what I was dreading, but I was still confident it wouldn't happen to me.

I was in the hospital for about a week after I started treatment. This was to see how I was coping with the treatment and to look for any side effects. It wasn't all that bad; one of the volunteers named Zach had come and hung out with me. He was an amazing man who helped and cheered up sick kids. I liked him a lot because he played the PlayStation with me. That's right, the kids' ward had a PlayStation. I always made sure to borrow one. You could play any game you wanted with the big TV on a wheelie cart. This got me through the first few days, but that's when the side effects started to hit. I am trying to think how I can make this not graphic, so apologies in advance but look, it has to be said, as I can't leave out any details now, can I?

Extreme nausea and vomiting ensued; I am talking about vomiting until nothing can come up anymore. The fatigue was next level as well; I just fell asleep and slept all day. My loving parents were always by my side though, forcing me to take showers and clean my bed, and even my stubborn father made me go for walks around the ward. Dad's insistence on making me go for stupid walks was a constant source of frustration, but it was necessary for me to stay active. So I guess, thanks, Dad; it definitely helped, but at the time, I was ropeable!

After the first round of chemotherapy, I was allowed to go home. This became a recurring thing that I would look forward to: being in my own house with my family. Sad to say, this wasn't a given, as any slight chance of an infection or sickness would mean that we would be straight back to the hospital. We had to check my temperature twice a day, morning and night, to ensure that it was never above 37.5 degrees. If it was, I was to come in. If I felt sick, I was to come in. If I felt any pain or weirdness, I was to come in. That was my rule set: any abnormalities were a hospital trip. This was especially challenging for us, as being such a young kid/family at the time, we were exposed to large numbers of nasty bugs and viruses. So this made staying away from infections almost impossible.

Goodbye, Hair

After the first cycle of chemotherapy treatment, I was back home and enjoying my comfy bed. One morning I remember waking up, and I could feel something itchy on the back of my neck. This was a concern for me, as here in Australia, a weird itchy feeling on your neck could mean one of many different things. At the top of the list of things that you don't want to make your neck itchy are spiders, creepy crawlies and all the rest. My initial reaction was to feel what it was, as anyone would really. Bracing for the worst, I instinctively picked up whatever was bothering me. Half expecting to brush away the nuisance, I found myself clutching strands of my own hair. It was a surreal moment, and I think this was the moment it actually all kind of hit me. Losing your hair is almost like losing a part of your identity.

At the time, this was all that was playing through my head. I attempted to verify this by running my hands through my hair, but each attempt resulted in additional loose hair. This is one of the times when I struggled to find my positive mindset. It really was a dark time; I felt embarrassed, naked and ashamed. These are all completely normal feelings, but I just wanted to be a kid. I was already feeling crook and tired; now the visible effects were setting in. I didn't want to go to school because my hair was falling out. Not only that, but I refused to get it wet or do anything to it as I wanted hold onto my hair a little while longer. Kind of like Homer Simpson with his two final strands of hair.

You can laugh; it's okay. I can laugh about it now, but it's how I felt at the time. However, as I mentioned earlier in the story, I had the support of family and friends, which helped reinforce my positive mindset and overall aided me when I was down. I have the best family and friends that I could possibly ask for. When I was feeling sorry for myself, they had other plans, and let me just tell you, it was one of the nicest gestures that I could've asked for. My school was supportive by bringing in guest speakers to explain to everyone what was going on with me and why I would be bald, etcetera. It was a lovely gesture, but at the same time, it made me feel a bit more scared because I thought everyone would easily identify me as the sick one due to my appearance.

Funnily enough, there weren't too many bald ten-year-old boys going around, so I just kept thinking, *I am going to stick out* and *people will notice me*. This is when, little to my knowledge, my family and friends had something planned that would help solve all of these problems. Let's just say there were going to be more than a few bald kids rocking up to school on Monday. You know what they say: bald is beautiful.

Let me introduce you to the people who willingly shaved off their luscious locks without a second thought to join me in being bald. Might I add that this was also September? So just coming off winter, it was still quite chilly this time of year. And let me tell you from first-hand experience, you feel the cold *a lot* more when you don't have any hair on your head. So next time you're making fun of your dad and grandpa or anyone really who you love and is bald, think about the struggles they have. Not just with the cold but also with the sun! Here are the boys who joined me, listed in no particular order:

Vaughan, Lachlan W, Jarvis, Reid, Kevin, Finley, Kai, Ashton, Marley.

I also can't forget about Dad, Steve, and his wonderful mate, whom I know as Jonno (Johnothan).

On a cold winter's morning, these boys joined me at LOXX salon, where a lovely lady by the name of Karen shaved all of our heads. These boys didn't want me to face this alone, so they all joined in solidarity, shaving their heads and becoming a bunch of eggheads. I will never be able to express my gratitude to these boys – massive shout-out to them. I was nervous about being the 'outsider' at school, but thanks to them, I didn't feel alone. One by one, we lined up and got our heads shaved all together. This was a wonderful morning, filled with laughs, as it was so funny. *I just have the best support,* I kept thinking to myself. Special shoutout to Lachy, who had gelled his hair that day and wasn't quite as eager to lose his hair, but he did it anyway (the girls liked you more without hair, mate).

It was such a special day for me, and I felt like I was not alone in this battle. After the haircuts were finished and all the photos were done, we headed off to school together to show off our new cuts. However, on the way home in the car, I started to feel a bit sick and fatigued. My mum and I made the executive decision to keep me at home, so unfortunately I missed out on seeing my teacher's face when everyone showed up without any hair. The boys did tell me that it was priceless, so I had to just go with that.

When I was up to it, the school visits would come. These were times when I could feel just like a kid and ignore the external things that were playing in the background of my life. The further I got in treatment, though, the less I was able to make it to school. Regular blood tests were a common necessity, as they had to monitor how my body was responding to treatment. They checked my blood cell counts to make sure my immune system stayed strong enough to fight infections and detected any early signs of complications. The tests also assessed how my liver and kidneys were handling the chemotherapy, ensuring the treatment wasn't causing more harm than good.

These frequent checks gave the doctors valuable information on whether my treatment was working and helped them adjust it as needed to keep me safe and on track. My white blood cell count was extremely low, so by this time public appearances were becoming scarcer. I didn't mind it though as I was able to get closer with my family, and my mates were always one text or phone call away. My cat Eddie was always looking after me as well. He was old, so he was always happy to lie down and just relax. This is all I was really doing at that point, so it was a win–win situation. It was also a time when I was in a positive headspace. I knew I was sick, but I was kind of oblivious to the unfolding situation as my parents kept me sheltered from all the terrible things that were happening. I knew I was very sick, but with the help of my parents, family and friends, I kept a positive attitude and just looked forward to when I was going to be back to my sports and exercises. October was the light at the end of the tunnel, so I just had to roll with the punches until then.

It took a bit before the hospital holidays and visits came, but when they did, they were never-ending. I used to try to keep a record of my longest stays. I am not sure who I was competing with, but I used to think of it as a competition with myself. One of my first overnight hospital stays was actually one of my most memorable, and not for a good reason at all. Not throwing shade at Mum at all, but I think this night took about twenty years off of her life, not even joking. It was one of the scariest nights of her and my life. I honestly think my whole family's life, as the night was intense, to say the least. Here it goes, so strap in, grab your popcorn and get ready for this. If I make this sound dramatic in any way, I am not apologising at all because it was. Trust me.

The night started off as normal as could be at the time. Mum was making maybe roast pork or cutlets, something along those lines. Pretty much my favourite foods to try and get me to eat. When you're undergoing chemotherapy, you often feel unwell and find it difficult to consume food. So you pretty much get spoiled in an attempt to get you to eat. I frequently found myself indulging in some pretty solid feeds. I had to take certain medications before meals; however, there were two types of pills that were the exact same medication but different milligrams of the medicine. I can't remember the exact amounts, but I am fairly sure it was 25 mg and 75 mg or something like that.

Mum was exhausted, as she always seemed to be back then – understandably stressed, trying to keep the other boys okay, all while constantly worrying about me. She got the pills out for me, and she accidentally – well, I hope it was! *Only kidding* – gave me two of the higher-dose pills, the 75 mg ones. I normally took one 75 mg in the morning or like twice 25 mg at night or something. Pretty much, Mum accidentally gave me double or triple the dose that I was meant to have. Now, with these medications I was on, just like the chemotherapies, they have a truckload of side effects. You can see how this was terrible, since too much of anything can be dangerous.

I took the tablets without a second thought and continued with my dinner. It was only when Mum got up to grab something from the bench that she realised the mistake she had made. She had taken out two boxes of the stronger tablet and given them to me. This is where things took a serious turn for the worse. Mum immediately started freaking out and telling Dad we had to take me to the hospital right now. In a scream, she explained what mix-up she had made, and that is when the house went into chaos.

Dad grabbed me and took me downstairs to start throwing up the delicious meal that we had just eaten. He was sticking his fingers down my throat to vomit up these tablets I had taken. I was so devastated about it, as it was a wonderful dinner. However, in such situations, you can't take any chances. The meal was so good that I don't think there were any leftovers. I am still upset about that to this day because it was such a nice dinner!

Mum was upstairs grabbing clothes for me to wear at the hospital as Dad and I were in the car. It was such a terrible night; I had kind of grasped what was going on, stressing I was going to die. Mum was upstairs hysterically crying, and Dad had got me in the car, speeding off to the hospital. The situation was truly distressing. Mum's friend Paula, who is a massive legend, came over to help. She has been a paramedic her whole life, and she's excellent in stressful situations. Dad was frantically calling people from the hospital, letting them know what was happening. We were trying to reach a registered nurse who oversaw all the cancer kids. She would know what to do. This was a difficult task, though, as it was around 8:30 at night.

Suddenly, Dad's phone rang as we sat there in the car, just the two of us. The whole mood shifted instantly; we both went dead quiet, waiting for the nurse on the other end to speak. In a calm, almost casual tone, she explained that while I had definitely taken more of the pills than I should have, it wasn't the disaster we'd imagined. 'Honestly,' she said, 'you'd have to take a lot more for it to be a real issue. Just head to emergency to be certain, but there's no need to panic; you're going to be fine.'

The relief in the car was palpable. We both exhaled at the same time, and it felt like the weight of the world had just lifted. The massive freakout was over. I wasn't on the brink of death, and while we still had to head to the emergency room to double-check, the worst of the panic had passed.

Even now, I still give Mum a hard time about how she tried to poison me. Although I laugh about it with Mum, she doesn't quite see the humour in it. I don't know why! As for Dad, I don't think he's ever fully recovered from frantically driving to the hospital. Look, I am no snitch, but I don't think he was driving the speed limit. But this is all alleged as I had my head in a vomit bag.

I'm pretty sure that night added a few grey hairs to both of their heads. Even though we laugh about it now, I think that scare will be something neither of them will ever quite forget.

The Starlight Room

The first twenty-eight days were done, and I now looked unmistakably like a cancer patient. From August to September, my appearance changed drastically. My head was completely bald, and when I looked at my reflection, my features appeared hollow and gaunt in some places. It was so odd as I was malnourished in some places but puffy in others, especially my face. The puffiness was the result of prednisone, a steroid I had to take as part of my treatment. My cheeks looked swollen, as round as the moon, giving me a strange sense of unfamiliarity every time I caught a glimpse of myself in the mirror. I couldn't even recognise myself, which is a strange thing to say, but I wasn't able to.

Prednisone wasn't like the steroids I had seen bodybuilders use, though. It didn't make me look strong or muscular; instead, it filled me with a kind of bloated feeling. I think prednisone was my old friend from my previous hospital visit that I accidentally took too much of. Anyway, it was no good, as it made my limbs feel heavier, and my face carried this strange, stretched tightness. My body felt foreign in ways I would have never thought in a million years.

But at the same time, part of me felt kind of cool. After all, this was a steroid, and there was something about the name that carried an aura of power. I'd been told prednisone was there to help me fight, to reduce the inflammation in my body as it waged war on the cancer inside. In a sense, this gave me a sense of strength, as if I had an unseen ally, one that was fighting back in its own unique manner, despite the fact that it caused me to appear more swollen than I had ever been before.

It was also around this time that I started to learn my way around the hospital. The two most common wards you would catch me on would be on level 2 of the Sydney Children's Hospital, Randwick. One of the wards was C2North and the other ward was C2West. The way I distinguished the difference between them was that C2West was for sleepovers (it was a ward cancer kids stayed on when they were inpatients) and C2North was for day visits (outpatient ward). However, in saying this, a quick day trip to C2North could also turn into a sleepover at C2West. Both of these wards, though, were lovely; everyone there was awesome and made you feel at home. The wards weirdly ended up becoming a safe haven to me, and it was kind of comforting as they always took such great care of you. I was extremely grateful for the days I could spend in C2North.

Both of the wards were also places that really helped to give me perspective, even to this day. I will never forget the stories I heard from some of the sick kids who were in the trenches beside me. I felt so lucky and fortunate that I only needed two months of chemotherapy. Kids were in there for leukaemia, brain tumours, bone tumours, and everything. You name it, a kid had it. I was ten years old, and I was honestly, at times, one of the oldest. Many of the patients had been receiving treatment for more than a year, I had come to learn. I was baffled at the time, given how much chemotherapy can affect you; after all, I'd experienced it firsthand!. There were even toddlers and babies.

It made me so sad to see these families going through what they had to endure. Even just looking around the ward, it would break my heart. Kids' heads were so swollen from tumours that their eyes looked like they would pop out. It's just not fair at all, is it? No one should ever have to go through that, and that's why so many wonderful people are dedicated to the work they do – to help support these kids in any way. The nurses and doctors in those wards are real-life superheroes, and they deserve all the credit they get, plus more.

After one long day in the hospital, I was at home trying to relax in my bed, feeling pretty fortunate to be out of the hospital for a change. But suddenly, I felt this excruciating pain in my back. It was unlike anything I had ever felt before, easily a ten out of ten. I couldn't sit still; I couldn't find a position that eased it. No matter what I tried, nothing worked. I was by myself in my room when I called out to Mum. This was terrible pain. Mum didn't even bother giving me Panadol; she just took me straight to the hospital. My mum could see the pain on my face and knew it was bad. We arrived at the emergency, and with my trusty gold card, we were straight through. The gold card was like the golden ticket that all kid cancer patients were given, and it allowed us to go straight through emergency. Just like in *Willy Wonka*, except instead of a chocolate factory tour, I got a first-class ticket to scans, needles and fluorescent lighting – not exactly the dream day out!

The pain was a side effect of one of the chemos I'd been on. They weren't quite sure which one as they all had pain as a side effect. They started trying everything they could to get me comfortable and in less pain. I was given every painkiller they had, starting from Nurofen, but it was like my body didn't care. Nothing helped. I was still in agony, with no sign of the pain stopping or slowing down. This continued until they finally administered me with fentanyl. It was like my pain then suddenly faded away. That's when the pain began to ease, and for the first time in what felt like hours, I could breathe again. I thought I'd be able to finally rest after that, but things took a turn. See, this is the issue here. That is when my memory started to fade out. But my mum was there, and she definitely had a story to tell after that.

Here is what went down according to Mum's recollection. This is where the real chaos started. Apparently, I decided that running around the hospital was the next logical step, and, to make things more interesting, I started stripping off all my clothes. Mum said it was like I was on some kind of mission, completely out of my mind, darting through the hallways with doctors and nurses chasing after me, trying to get me back into bed. She told me I was running around like a headless chook, totally unaware of how ridiculous I looked.

It's one of those moments that, looking back, is hilarious, and we can have a good laugh about it. That said, my poor mum was probably horrified at the time. However, she did say that it was good to see me happy and smiling again, even if I was naked in the emergency department. It's quite funny how these things play out occasionally. I woke up the next morning having zero idea of what had taken place overnight. As soon as I was apparently done running around, I passed out. They kept me in C2West for several nights, solely for monitoring purposes. The next morning, I had to relive the entire saga through stories from the nurses and my family about what I got up to. Needless to say, I stayed in emergency overnight, and not long after, I was moved up to the C2West ward, where I spent the next few nights. It was one of those experiences that becomes more amusing the further away you get from it!

This stay only ended up being a few long days, but it was just one of the many times that I was in C2West. My friends would come and visit me when they could, which was always a positive time for me. It helped me to feel normal, like a kid again. That social aspect was an important thing for me, as I was such an outgoing kid. However, there was always the isolation that I felt. My friends had to keep their distance from me to avoid potentially making me sick. I also hated when people treated me differently or looked at me with sympathy. I always felt that I would be okay and that this was just a small hiccup in the grand scheme of things. Not only that, but I constantly looked towards the future; that was my coping mechanism. 'This will be horrible for now, but in a few months' time you will be all good,' this constantly echoed in my mind. I had an end-of-treatment date: October. The number of kids I met without an end date was horrifying. Imagine you didn't have one? What would your hope be?

There also were times in the Sydney kids' ward that really haunted me, and still do to this day. One of those times was when I was in C2West. I remember sitting in the hospital room, the sterile smell of antiseptic lingering in the air, a constant reminder of where we were. Across from me lay a kid in a bed, his pale face as white as a ghost. I couldn't shake the feeling that something was off. His mum sat by his side, her expression a mix of worry and helplessness, her eyes darting between the monitors and her son. She held his hand tightly, as if that simple act could somehow transfer her strength to him. It was so sad, as the boy's mum reminded me of my own. Knowing my mum, that lady would've done anything to trade places with her son, as would mine.

Then, the atmosphere shifted abruptly. A sense of urgency filled the room as they called in the resuscitation team. I watched in horror as nurses rushed in, their faces set in serious expressions, their movements quick and purposeful, all with intent. It was like watching a scene from a movie, but this was all too real. I was asked to step out and go to the Starlight

Room; I could tell something serious was going on, but due to my age, no one wanted to fill me in.

I entered the Starlight Room – the familiar purple glow, beanbags scattered like clouds and gaming consoles stretching as far as the eye could see usually made it a kid's paradise. Inside, I tried to keep my mind occupied, as it was a happy place for me, but all I could think about was the kid across the way and the commotion that was just happening. I played video games and tried to talk to other kids, but I was worried about that boy. After what felt like an eternity, we were finally allowed to return. As we walked back, I felt a mix of nervousness and hope, but the air was thick with an unshakeable tension.

When we entered the room, my heart sank. The bed was gone, leaving the space empty and haunting. Only his mum remained, gathering the last of their belongings. I could see her trembling hands as she packed up the last of the few items left behind. This highlighted the fact that they had to leave quickly. She was on the phone, her voice strained and cracking as she mentioned 'ICU'. The weight of those letters hung in the air. It felt like a punch to the gut. Where there had been life and worry just hours before, there was now an eerie silence. I will never forget this day.

I lay in my bed, trying to grapple with the reality of what had just happened. The sight of his empty bed and the sound of her quiet sobs were haunting reminders of the fragility of life. At that moment, I realised how quickly things could change. The weight of the situation pressed down on me, and

I felt a rush of emotions, including sadness, fear and a profound sense of helplessness. It was a moment that would forever be etched in my memory, a reminder of the battles fought within those sterile walls and the lives forever altered by this horrific circumstance. This is something that I have taken with me my whole life. I never found out what happened to that boy, but I hope that he is okay now and pulled through. We were all a team in there, and although we never spoke, I was rooting for him.

Music became a way to help me deal with the harshness of being a cancer patient, with Avicii being the leading artist I kept listening back to. Back then, I listened to a lot of music, but especially him. His song 'Wake Me Up' was my favourite as it felt like he understood me. The lyrics really spoke to me; I felt invincible and like it would all be over soon whenever the song was on. For that reason, I'll always have a special place in my heart for Avicii, and I'm grateful for him. It is funny how music can make such a big impact in people's lives. Avicii's music certainly helped me and still continues to do so.

As I mentioned earlier, the Starlight Room was something I looked forward to when I had my hospital visits in C2West. A group of volunteers ran a gaming room where kids from all over the hospital could come and hang out. It was such a wonderful initiative, and it made the hospital more enjoyable and less stressful. When I had the energy and permission, I would spend time playing games in the hospital. This helped to pick up the mood, and it allowed me to socialise with kids and feel like a normal ten year old. The best part about the

Starlight Room was that you didn't always have to be there to feel included; the weekly quiz was a great aspect that kept you socialising and feeling included, all from your hospital bed.

Every week, without fail, the quiz would kick off with the same song, 'Classic' by MKTO. It was one of those tunes that just got stuck in your head, not in a terrible way, but because you'd heard it a thousand times. As soon as the first beat dropped, you knew it was quiz time. It became, almost like clockwork, a kind of signal to get involved. And even though I wasn't always the biggest fan of the song, it's one of those things you end up attaching memories to, like an inside joke you never planned on.

I can still picture it: the music playing while we all gathered, ready for the quiz to start. It was the anthem of those nights, and hearing it felt like hitting 'play' on the same scene every week. That song was everywhere, filling the space before the first question was asked, calling us all together like a rallying cry. Even if we were tired or distracted, that tune would bring us back to the moment, like a little jolt reminding us that there was still some positivity in the surrounding circumstances.

It's funny how much a song can stick with you. 'Classic' became the soundtrack to that part of my life. It wasn't a song I would've chosen myself, but over time it just fit. Every time I hear it now, it takes me right back to those moments. It's woven into my mind, tied to the laughter, the friendly competition and the routine of those quiz nights.

I would grab the phone next to my bed and be waiting for the intro to conclude so the quiz could start. You would tell them your room and bed number so that if you were to either win or place, a prize would be hand-delivered to you. It was so cool, and no matter how sick or down I was feeling, I always made sure to participate in the quiz. Each week, another patient would create a quiz for everyone to participate in. They would get to go up to the film booth and present the quiz with one of the Starlight volunteers. I was so excited because I believed that it would be such an exciting and awesome experience, and I had plenty of time, I thought to myself. This is how the Shark quiz idea came to life.

Great White or Bull Shark?

I had an opportunity to pick one of my interests and turn it into a quiz. I can't exactly remember why I was so fascinated by sharks, but I loved them as a kid. Maybe it was because of the Cronulla Sharks, once again the best NRL team in the competition. Dad always promised me that when I was out of the hospital, we would swim to Shark Island (yes, there is a place in Cronulla called Shark Island) and go looking for sharks. Anyway, back to the infamous shark quiz. I told the Starlight volunteers I wanted to make a quiz, and they were excited because they had never done one with sharks as the top. I got all the nurses and doctors involved, even getting myself my whiteboard to draft up ideas and write interesting facts about sharks.

I spent days working on this project and learned everything I needed to know about the topic. I wish I could still remember certain facts, but I can tell you this: I believed that apparently bull sharks were the most dangerous sharks, even more than the great white. This was the perfect distraction as well, as the rounds of chemo kept coming, and I was able to divert my attention from the toxic substances in my body. Keeping distracted at that time was perfect, and I highly recommend it to others. Focusing on other tasks can sometimes help distract your mind from the harsh reality that's unfolding. Not too much, as you sometimes need to face the fire, but just enough. October was coming up, and that was when my treatment was going to end. Things like the shark quiz helped me to feel more normal and get back to doing schoolwork and research tasks.

The day I had been waiting for had arrived. It was time to present the quiz and show the hard work that I had put into it. I was to join Captain Starlight in the TV booth and get ready to present the PowerPoint. I got dressed up in my Cronulla Sharks beanie, and I was good to go. I was wheelchaired up to the Starlight Room as walking became a difficult task for me the longer treatment went on. We took the elevator up to Level 3, and it was showtime. I met Captain Starlight, and we were in the booth getting ready to go live. I still get goosebumps thinking about this moment as it was so awesome! I was given my microphone and the countdown was on until we were live. My heart was pounding I was so nervous, but also excited as I had put so much effort into the quiz.

The phone calls kept ringing, with many kids eager to play the quiz. It was so much fun, and everyone seemed to enjoy it!

Everyone did a lot better than I thought they would have. But I did stump them all with the question, Which shark is the most aggressive? Funnily enough, that's really the only slide I remember out of the whole quiz, as it had a photo of four different types of sharks.

Now, I will question you guys reading this: What is the most aggressive shark? Is it:

A: Great White
B: Bull Shark
C: Tiger Shark
D: Grey Nurse
E: Cronulla Sharks

I know you all think the answer is E, but it is in fact B, the bull shark. This stumped everyone, as they all thought it was the great white shark. Unfortunately, no one picked the Cronulla Sharks. I wonder why?

After it was all said and done, I thanked Captain Starlight for being the perfect cohost to my crazy quiz. I believe it was a great success, and if there is anyone who remembers participating in a shark quiz in the Sydney Children's Hospital in 2013, please feel free to reach out and give me a review. Just quickly as well, massive shoutout to the Starlight Foundation for all they do for the kids at the hospital. It made the hospital that little bit more bearable, and for that, thank you guys.

Another great memory from the Starlight Room was meeting Timomatic, the Australian singer. That was an awesome experience, and thank you very much for organising that, and for Timomatic for taking the time out of his day to visit us. It really makes you realise that there is so much good in this world, and at the time of writing this, I look back at it with a smile, and that is only due to the hard work that these volunteers put in.

At last, my final chemotherapy treatment was put on the drip. It was a surreal day, and this short celebration was also one of great consequence as I had to get a PET scan after this to see if there were any signs of cancer left. The two months of consistent treatment felt like a lifetime, and if all was well, it was coming to an end. It all felt like a weird dream, to be honest. All the hospital admissions and everything all just kind of blurred into one big nightmare. So nothing really was special about the day; we went home and had a nice dinner, but we kind of just enjoyed the peace. As of these past two months, that was a foreign thing to my family and me. The date was set for the PET scan, which was to be on the 3rd of October. This was, at the time, the most important day of my life.

There were only two outcomes of the PET scan. Option 1: the cancer is all gone, and I can finally move on with my life. Or Option 2: there is still visible cancer. If treatment didn't work, I would have to undergo further treatment, including radiation therapy. The longer that treatment goes on, the higher the chance for terrible side effects and, overall, a worse prognosis. Also, radiotherapy would have been used, which has very severe side effects, but unlike chemotherapy, they are mostly long-term and much more catastrophic, such as secondary cancers. It was kind of do or die; we put all our faith and trust in Toby, and we followed everything he had said.

The day had arrived, for my final PET scan. I remember following all the procedures like I had done before, drinking all the liquid and staying warm. I felt like I was professional at this now as I could generally do this with my eyes closed. Although, I didn't experience the normal anxious feeling that I'm sure everyone else was experiencing. I trusted the process. Clinically, my lymph nodes on my neck, which were once tennis balls, were much smaller. Almost normal size, which was where my confidence came from. 'Your lymph nodes will always have scarring,' I was always told, so in saying that, I was in quite a good mindset and ready for the last push of the journey. The 45-minute scan flew by then it was all finished. Now it was just the waiting game for the appointment so Toby could tell us what was next.

It was only a few days later when we were back in C2North, this time in Toby's office, about to get news that could drastically change the course of my life. I walked with my head up high, no cords attached to me anymore through my portacath, which was a great feeling. Now I can't lie, I was still so nervous that it almost didn't feel real. It was the day we had all been waiting for. We walked in, and Toby greeted me with his familiar 'Hi Maestro' with a big smile on his face. This wasn't any different, so we didn't want to get our hopes up. Just like that horrific day a few months ago, both Mum and Dad came into the appointment today. Usually it would just be one of them with me, but due to the magnitude of the moment, they both came.

The best thing about Toby is that he is direct and straight to the point. Sometimes this could be a scary concept, but on a day like this, it was what we needed. And just like that, with a smile on his face, he exclaimed the words, 'Clear PET scan, no signs of cancer.' It was the single greatest thing that I have ever heard. After those rough few months, it had all come to an end. My parents cried with joy and were hugging me. It was such an awesome day, and I will never forget it.

We thanked Toby greatly, with many hugs and praises, and we might have even given him some chocolates, if I remember correctly. They weren't Cadbury chocolates, but rather a delightful assortment of homemade chocolates. We left C2North that day, happy as can be. All the side effects and everything we'd endured were so worth it, just for this moment. Toby still wanted us to do check-ups every three months for the first eighteen months, then every six months for the next year, and finally yearly after that. As much as I loved seeing Toby, it was nice to hear that I wouldn't be seeing him too much anymore. No offence to Toby, of course!

Now this is quite funny, actually; we left that day with smiles on our faces, feeling unstoppable, ready to take on the world. However, a day or two later, we found ourselves back in the hospital as I had obtained a slight temperature, which meant a trip to the emergency room. It is hilarious now that I think about it, as we'd said our big goodbyes to everyone for now, and I was back in such a short period. I was all okay, just a slight infection, so I used my trusty gold pass to get straight through the emergency, and I was back to C2West.

More Needles

On the first night I was back in hospital, I remember the hospital room I was in being dim, sort of mysterious with not much light covering the room, allowing for shadows to smother. I was in bed waiting for the nurse to come in and tell us what was going on. The PET scan was clear, and we had just had the best news ever. We were still cheering and counting our blessings, considering that grave day in August 2013 was now seemingly well past us. It was now October, and I was finished with treatment, just having a small vacation in the hospital. However, something was off. My portacath had stopped working. Nurses could no longer draw blood from it or put liquids through it anymore. There was a clog somewhere. This was quite normal for the ports, as the longer they sit in there, the more the body recognises it as a foreign object and creates a barrier inside of it.

TWICE BEFORE TWELVE

This wasn't a concern for anyone involved, until someone spotted something foreign on my PET scan. A dark-coloured shape ingrained in my internal jugular vein. I was just minding my own business when a nurse walked in to tell us the bad news. I was told I was going to be taking a blood thinner known as clexane for over three months. This was two needles, morning and night, to help treat the blood clot and ensure that it didn't spread anywhere. It was a scary thing to process, as the function of the internal jugular vein is to collect blood from the skull, brain, superficial parts of the face, and the majority of the neck. In layman's terms, essentially it is a crucial vein, and mine was completely clogged up. I was heartbroken to learn that I could not participate in any contact sports due to the risk of severe bleeding and bruising. Which would not be good at all, to say the least.

Although this news was annoying, I stopped for a second and pondered. For a while, I couldn't get back to all the old sports and activities I loved, but I was grateful for my health. I reflected on all the kids I'd met on this horrendous but short journey and thought of them. This helped me to see the bright side of the situation. *I have survived cancer; a few little needles in my stomach each day are nothing. It won't be forever; it is just short-term. There is always light at the end of the tunnel. No matter how dire a situation may seem, there is always something to be grateful for and hopeful about.* I couldn't do much exercise, but I could get good at FIFA on the PlayStation. I'd lost all my hair, so I got to try a new haircut and see what I looked like bald. This experience might be more helpful as I age, though.

Life can suck, and things can make you feel terrible, whether that be relationships, injuries, sicknesses or whatever it may be. But with a change of mindset, you can drastically prohibit these things from getting to you and making you feel worse. As I was always told as a kid, 'It's good to stop and smell the roses sometimes.' This mindset, even as a ten year old, helped me endure the painful clexane injections. They were such a punishment for two reasons. The first reason was because they felt like a bee sting. The stinging sensation was the worst, which is all that needs to be said. The second reason was, as I was so skinny, to find fat on my body was an impossible task. The needle had to be injected into fat stores, so it was either your bum or stomach. Look, I wasn't a big fan of my mum or dad putting a needle in my buttocks' region, so the stomach it was.

The clexane was very annoying but luckily I was allowed to go away to my Year 4 camp at Waterslea. I could participate in ninety per cent of the activities, and in my eyes, it was the perfect celebration for me after the last three months that I'd had to endure. Dad came along with me, and I believe he truly enjoyed spending time with my teachers as they appeared to be having a wonderful time.

For the time being, my cancer journey seemed to be concluded, and everything seemed to be going smoothly – as if I would lead a happy and fulfilling life. Or so we thought.

TWICE BEFORE TWELVE

Friday, 25th October 2013, 21:35:00 Trisha Cashmere <t*******cashmere**@gmail.com>wrote:

Subject: *Update on Angus*

Hi Everyone,

After spending most of the school holidays in hospital, we received some great news after Angus' first round of post-treatment scans: **"No identifiable active cancer."** (Collective sigh of relief.) Importantly, this means no radiotherapy at this time. There will be PET and CT scans every three months for the next 18 months, just to make sure everything stays on track.

Angus' immunity will continue to be compromised for around 3–6 months, and I haven't yet told him that the chemo has probably "undone" all of his childhood immunisations, so he has that to look forward to.

Angus has developed a clot in his internal jugular vein, probably a consequence of the portacath. This means twice daily injections of clexane and no physical activity that poses a risk of a bump or bang because of the associated increased propensity to bleed until January 4th, 2014. This is frustrating for Angus (and for those of us who are a bit horrified at sticking needles in someone), but it's temporary. Overall, we feel that we've gotten through this relatively lightly (although Angus may not agree with that assessment!).

Angus is currently campaigning hard to go on the Year 4 camp to Waterslea in late November. We are trying to make it happen, and his medical team is on board. Either Steve or I will also be attending if Angus gets to go. I recall that 11 was my favourite age ever, so reliving it for a bit might be okay.

We are slowly getting back to what I'm thinking of as a new normal. It will take some time, but there's no rush. I'm personally working hard on overcoming my tendency to tear up unexpectedly (it's so weird, and it gets embarrassing at Woolies...).

Thank you all for your support throughout this experience. Knowing that so many of you care for us and our son(s) has made this journey that much easier to navigate. I look forward to seeing each of you in the near future.

As with previous emails, feel free to pass this on as you see fit. Hopefully, this will be my last update about Angus and cancer. I'm looking forward to letting you all know about the wonderful life he will make for himself in the years to come. Much love and endless thanks, Trish

Intermission

My portacath removal surgery was scheduled for November 6th 2013, a quick 45-minute procedure. It's quite ironic when you consider that, despite all the complexities and challenges of cancer treatment, removing the port was such a quick and straightforward process. Physically, all that remained afterwards was a scar about six centimetres long on my right pec, and a few smaller ones behind my ear and on my neck. These scars have become much more than a mark. They stand as a lasting reminder of the fight I'd endured over the past three months, a symbol of the battles I've faced, things that I will carry with me for the rest of my life.

I wrapped up the clexane in early January 2014 and it was go time. Even though I still secretly skateboarded behind my parents' back the whole time I was on the blood thinner (sorry, guys), I was now off it and ready to take on the world. This was perfect timing to discontinue the clexane, as it was just in time for our annual trip down the south coast to Narooma. My family has been going there for years, meeting up with our cousins and having the best time. Narooma is a breathtaking coastal location, about a 4.5-hour drive from Sydney. This was and still is my family's happy place, so you could imagine how excited we were to get away for over a week and relax.

I was now starting Year 5, and I had one thing on my mind, and that was rugby league. I would practise in the yard for hours, trying to catch every bomb and every grubber. The year before, I played in the De La Salle Caringbah A2's side. They were the second-best team. I was so committed to making the A1 side, which was the top side; it was my goal. When I was sick, it was literally all I could think about. Footy trials came, and my name was announced in the top team, the A1s. I was so excited; after all the hardship of the year prior, I was finally back to doing what I loved, and I hadn't skipped a beat at all, or no one could tell at least.

In June 2014, my parents embarked on an unforgettable journey around the Northern Territory. It was the perfect trip to move past the horrors that we'd faced last year. I think it gave my whole family a new look on life and how precious it is. I think to them, it was a celebration for us all, which was such a wonderful idea. The whole family was very shaken by my cancer journey. What better way to reflect on that while travelling through Australia's most dangerous territory, due to the heat and the animals? The place is full of snakes, crocodiles, spiders, and you name it; I can guarantee they are lurking there. Even the weather wants to kill you. All jokes aside, it is such a breathtaking place, and it was the perfect idea for the family to get closer.

The trip involved us setting off on a big adventure that Mum and Dad planned out. Dad had just completed the Shitbox Rally, which is a great charitable foundation. It involves a team of people driving cars worth under $1500 across Australia in some of the harshest environments. The Shitbox Rally is a great initiative, and they raise lots of money for cancer patients. Dad and his good mate Rob Hoy both participated in the event. The car they drove was named 'Angus & the Beefcakes' after me. Get it? My name is Angus, Angus Beef. It was a satirical name, which we all thought was funny. We planned to complete it in Darwin that year, which is why we chose to spend our holiday there.

The plan was to hire a six-person motorhome and to drive around the Northern Territory for around a month. We set off on the 5th of June 2014 for Darwin Airport and went from feeling trapped in hospital rooms to exploring the outback in just over eight months. Crazy, am I right?

Now, I need to quickly give some context regarding my family holidays. So, most families will go on a nice, relaxing beach holiday or something along these lines. However, not my family; my parents' (dad's) idea of holidays always involves a level of strenuous exercise. On this holiday, we had a trip booked where we would be kayaking down the Kathryn River and camping on the riverbanks. This was all fun and games until you learned that the Katherine River was home to the notorious Australian saltwater crocodile.

You may remember from before that I was quite a fan of sharks. This did not, in fact, carry through to crocodiles. I was scared to death of those things. Crocodiles were one of my biggest fears the whole trip, and I didn't want to go near the water or anything. Even in places considered 'safe' for swimming by Australian standards, I remained hesitant. I didn't want myself or any members of my family to end up as dinner for a large crocodile. You also couldn't swim on the beaches because there were box jellyfish, which are the world's most deadly jellyfish. The Northern Territory is incredible. I hope that I haven't scared anyone off at all as I will definitely be going back.

I have a few highlights from the holiday, which I think you guys will all enjoy, so here we go: One is quite simple, just cycling around Uluru. It is honestly one of the most beautiful places in Australia, and I would highly recommend anyone to go see it. The indigenous Dreamtime stories, too, just make the place magical. The entire Northern Territory is beautiful, filled with rich history and stunning landscapes.

The Crazy Bird. Yes, that is correct, a crazy bird has made the highlight list. I need to establish the scene first.

I remember this as a horror movie, and look, I may be being a little bit dramatic, but I need to tell it in that context for everyone to understand what we went through. It all started on a dark and stormy night. I am just kidding; it was a scorching hot day.

We were walking along the trail near the Glenn Helen Resort and all of a sudden we found a galah. This galah was like none that we had ever encountered in our lives. It was (seemingly) friendly – well, to Dad, at least. The galah landed on Dad's shoulder and stayed there as we were walking. It was so cool; we were all amazed at the bird as usually Australian animals are shy. We snapped some photos of Dad with it, and that is when we tried to get it to go on another one of our shoulders.

I tried to go first and let it go on my shoulder, but the thing kept trying to bite my ear or finger. It eventually nipped me, but Mum and Dad thought I was just carrying on. Everyone attempted to persuade the bird to perch on their shoulders, but it preferred to remain on Dad's.

When it did, however, get to other people's shoulders, it would bite them. When I said nip before, that was an understatement; this bird would fully bite you. On the ear or on the finger, whatever, it wouldn't stop! It got to the point where we were pretty fed up with the thing and were trying to ditch it. I can't remember who exactly, but one of the boys actually drew blood from the bite. That's when we realised that the bird was not leaving us alone.

Dad tried to put the galah down; however, it kept on flying back to his shoulder. Mum would try to get it off Dad's shoulder, but it would bite her. The thing was a deadset MENACE. The bird continued to follow us and no matter how many times we shooed it away, it wouldn't leave us alone. My brothers and I started running away from it, with Henry even locking himself in an outdoor dunnie (toilet for any non-Aussies) to get away. The galah landed on the roof, and Henry later explained that it felt like a scene from a horror movie. 'I could hear its sharp claws scraping against the tin roof.' He was happy to lock himself in there and not worry about the rest of us boys! We called the hike short and started to make our way out of the bush to try and escape the grasp of this bloody galah.

The end of the trail was near, and the galah had flown off – we'd completely lost sight of it. We finally reached the highway, where some people stopped to see why we were panting and what was going on. We were explaining to the lovely people what we had just endured from this pesky galah when we heard a quite familiar noise. The flapping of wings, then thuds, like gentle taps, as its sharp claws contacted the metal of the car. It had found us again, and it was deadset back! This thing was possessed. I am not even joking.

The galah had found a new partner, as it moved onto the man's shoulder we had just met. Now, we are generally a nice family, but in this situation, it was every man for himself, so we left the galah with the strangers. If you guys are reading this, we are sorry, but it had to be done. Such an eventful day, but hey, it's a timeless story to look back on.

Another highlight would've had to have been the NSW State of Origin win. We were staying in a caravan park, and I made a bet with Dad that if the Blues won, to celebrate, I would run around the park in my underwear and nothing else. Look, I don't know what my obsession was with always stripping off my clothes as a kid, but at least it was funny, right?

I am sure you can guess what happened next: the Blues won, and it was up to me to fulfil my bet. As promised, I undressed and sprinted around the caravan park. It was hilarious, especially since most of the guests were Queenslanders. I definitely felt that I represented the New South Welshman reputation well.

All up, the Northern Territory trip was one of the greatest experiences of my life. My brothers and I got closer, and it was the perfect holiday that we all needed. We had a great time, and no one was eaten by a crocodile or any of the other deadly animals there, so a successful trip to say the least. We learned all about the rich history of Australia before colonisation and met many wonderful people along the way. I distinctly sensed that the challenging year had come to an end, and we were embarking on an exciting journey ahead. I also remember losing heaps of teeth on that trip. I can confirm that the tooth fairy made it to the Northern Territory, so I was cheering.

Life Goes On

After our incredible journey, it was time to return to our regular routine. We continued on with our three-monthly check-ups with Toby. He was thrilled with how I had been progressing as my fitness levels were back, and I was putting weight back on. He had even pushed our check-ups to every six months, as clinically I was doing very well. Toby also said that if the cancer was going to reoccur, it would be in my neck again, so we would be able to tell if my lymph nodes became extremely enlarged again. This was fantastic news, as we eagerly anticipated seeing less of Toby (with all due respect, of course). It felt wonderful to start looking and feeling like myself again with the sunken-in sick look slowly fading away. I was coming back and it felt incredible.

This was around the time that my grandfather Barry 'Baz' Cunningham passed away at the age of seventy-nine. He was a great man who taught me to stand up for myself and for what is right. We got a call one morning from my Nanna Mary saying that Baz had had a fall and was not well. Dad immediately got in the car and drove up to go and see him in Laurieton, about an hour outside of Port Macquarie. We were on standby because we didn't realise the severity of the situation; we assumed he would be okay. Not even an hour and a half after Dad left, he called us and told us that we needed to come up and say goodbye, as the situation was dire. We all got into the car and drove as quickly as we could. The drive was around four and a half hours from my house, so we didn't have time on our hands.

When we got there, Baz was not well at all. I didn't really comprehend that he was dying; I just hoped and assumed he was going to get better because that's what hospitals do. They did it for me. Baz would always ring me after my hospital appointments to check in and see how I was doing. I remember Christmas 2013, when he made a special announcement for me at the dinner table to all our family and friends, saying he was proud of me beating cancer that year. He was my best mate. At the hospital, Mum tried to tell us as much as she could without upsetting us, but she did let us know that we had to say goodbye. I will never forget walking into the room and seeing him with all the tubes coming out of his mouth and other medical equipment. I will never forget the sight of this strong man, whom I admired, looking so sick. We spent the night with him, just saying how much we loved him and appreciated him. I held his hand for the last hour, and all I could think about was how cold it was; it didn't feel like Bazza. We left the hospital late that night after our goodbyes, which was the last time I ever saw him alive.

We visited him again in the hospital the morning he passed for a few final goodbyes, and that is when it all hit me. I was so distraught; I couldn't believe he was gone. His funeral was one of the hardest days of my life, as I opted to speak. I barely got a word out between my cries, with the only thing I mumbled being that 'he was my best mate'. Rest in peace, Baz. I hope you're enjoying a Guinness and watching the cricket up there.

Before I carry on with my story, I just want to mention my favourite memory of Bazza to show the type of man he was: the traditional Australian larrikin who didn't take crap from anyone. Baz taught me and my brothers how to play cricket. I remember one Christmas at their place in Laurieton, we got a cricket set for Christmas. Baz would bowl my older brother Henry and me balls while we batted. Each time he threw a ball, we would smack it, and it would ricochet all around the house. My nanna would tell us to stop as we were going to break something, but Baz couldn't contain his laughter and he kept on doing it. We were all cracking up as occasionally he'd let out a swear word, and Nanna would get more agitated, but he kept doing it. He was a great man, and I hope I make him proud every day. Love you, Baz.

Footy season was upon us, and I was ready to show my new team what I was made of. I was surprisingly fit still, but the only thing that lacked was my tackling (defence). I remember my coach keeping me back a few training sessions and getting the big boys to keep running at me until I could tackle them. This was the old way of doing it, but it eventually helped, as I ended up loving tackling. My technique only grew better, and I ended up peaking at eleven years old. I wish I had peaked a bit later, but look, I am grateful that I ever got to play my best footy, especially after what I'd endured the year before.

The season was going well for us, and we even got the opportunity to play Ipswich in a club versus club game. I ended up scoring a hat trick that game, which I was so stoked about. This is particularly evident when you consider the size difference between us and those Queensland boys. They looked years older than us, being much bigger and stronger than us, but funnily enough, we ended up smashing them.

We beat pretty much every team in the competition, but there was one team, our rivals, that we lost to. They had beaten us, and we had beaten them. Gymea also ended up being the minor premiers, finishing on top of the ladder. Both us and Gymea were beating every team that we came up against, so it was only inevitable that we met them in the big dance (Grand Final).

The day had come, almost a year ago to the date I was diagnosed with cancer, and now a year later I was in my first rugby league grand final. I was back! I felt completely normal and ready to put my body on the line for my team. The game was locked in: 11A De La Salle JRLFC vs. Gymea Gorillas JRLFC at Shark Park. All my family came down to support me: my grandparents, uncles, you name it, they were there. Once again, I'm just portraying the amount of support that I've had around me my whole life. I'm truly grateful!

It was a very close game, with little to no score in it at all. Unfortunately, I didn't get a touch of the ball nearly as much as I would've liked. You could definitely tell that it was the two best teams going back and forth. We scored first and converted the goal. Gymea then followed up with their own try, equalising the score at 6–6. There were many close moments where Gymea almost scored, and we were all starting to get nervous as momentum had shifted. We scored the final try and won the game, 12–6. I still smile when I think about it now; it was such an unforgettable experience. The bench stormed the field, and we all jumped around and celebrated like it was New Year's Eve. The best part was that the last thing on my mind was the horrific previous year. Likewise with my family, everything was going so well. In fact, 2014 was such a great year. We had a wonderful trip, I won a grand final and it seemed as though we were finally getting some good luck.

Year 5 at my primary school was also the time when you nominated yourself to become a school leader, being the captain or prefect. This was based on a voting system, where kids from Year 3 up to Year 5 all get to vote for who they want to represent the school. Being the extrovert I am, with no hesitation, I applied for the role. It was a long process where you have to give speeches. To even be eligible, the application has to be accepted by the teacher in charge of student leaders. I had many friends and got along with a lot of people, so I was hopeful that my luck would continue this year, and I would get a leadership position. I always had my sights set on becoming school captain, even though I told others that just being a prefect would be incredible. Deep down, I was really aiming for the top spot. I was also lucky that my younger brother Noah was in Year 3 so that he could get his friends to vote for me.

The first round of voting went through, and fortunately, I had made it through! It felt so good telling my parents this. Just seeing the smile on their faces made me feel happy, as I had become used to seeing them upset or crying around me. I know it's not my fault, but still, seeing people who care so much about you so devastated, it takes a toll on you. So to make it through the first round of voting was such a surreal moment; I had only advanced past the first round, and they were so excited. This was all the motivation I needed to try to go all the way and become the school captain. I brainstormed ways to win, and this is what I came up with: The key to winning the, let's say, 'election' for school leadership was the teacher's vote. Their vote carried more weight than a typical student's vote. I am not going to say that I was sucking up to my teachers, but I'll say that I was definitely over nice. I'm just joking (kind of); I always strived to be a nice and polite kid. Most of my reports would back this, with the only negative comment deadset being that I never stop talking. Who would believe that?

After the first round of nominations, the candidates and I had to do a speech in front of the whole school to say why they should vote for us. Looking back, the speeches were actually of good quality, with a few of the classic hilarious 'Coke in the bubblers' promises being thrown around a few times. Look, promising Coke in a bubbler in Year 5 was the key to victory. I remember my speech; I just wanted to keep it honest and true to myself. I wanted everyone to vote for the real me, not sell a fake story of why I would be a successful leader.

My speech performed significantly better than I had anticipated. I was always good at public speaking, but persuading people to trust you as a leader is different. I could see a few people in the crowd nodding along, which was either a positive sign or they were just trying to stay awake. Who knows! As previously mentioned, I maintained a realistic approach, refraining from making extravagant promises such as complimentary lunches or additional holidays, and simply being myself. When I wrapped it up, I had that feeling you get when you've done a half-decent job, like people actually appreciated it. Now, all that was left was the awkward waiting period, where you pretend you're not obsessively thinking about the outcome but secretly every night it's the only thing on your mind.

Ballots were distributed to all eligible students after the candidates had finished their speeches. Each student could vote for their preferred candidate by writing a number from 1 to 5 next to the corresponding name on the ballot paper. Candidates could vote for themselves number 1, so I had to do that for myself. They used our school photos on the piece of paper, and I couldn't help but reflect on mine. It was so different from anyone else's as the photo was taken at the start of the year when I had not much hair. I stared at the picture for a little bit; I had been so caught up in everything but now the past was well behind me. My fake smile conveyed a powerful message as I attempted to maintain a brave demeanour amidst the challenges of my life. Then I smiled, thinking about all my accomplishments until now; nothing could stop me and never was ever going to.

The way in which we found out we were going to be school leaders was by an announcement from the principals, but you didn't know whether you were a prefect or a school/vice-captain. Not until the day of the leadership assembly would you find out what your role was going to be. I remember the day that I found out I was a school leader; I was so proud. I was filled with immense joy and prepared to fully represent both my peers and my school. I didn't know what leader I was quite yet, but I knew that whether a prefect or captain, I was going to be present and ready to undertake any given task. It was funny; the year prior I missed so much school, but I was jokingly saying to my parents how I couldn't miss any school next year, with the opportunity I was given as a leader. Once again, who would've thought? My parents were so proud of me, and I called up every family member to tell them the great news. It all just showed the type of kid I was: resilient.

If you had just met me, you would've had no idea of what I had endured. I liked it. It was proof to me that one moment in life doesn't define you. Instead it's the actions you take afterwards that do.

The leadership ceremony was coming up, and soon I was going to find out what position I would hold in 2015. The ceremony involved the current leaders pinning the badges on the up-and-coming cohort, which was my year. I was good mates with the school captain at the time, so I was hoping that he was going to be the one to put the pin on me. Partly because I genuinely wanted to be school captain – and partly because it felt like one of those unforgettable moments, like a symbolic passing of the torch.

We all had to make speeches once we knew our allocated roles in front of the whole school. Both Mum and Dad came to watch the assembly and see what my role was. It felt like Christmas; the day had finally arrived. This was one of the most important days of my primary school career. I loved my school, and more than anything, I wanted to represent it – especially after all the support they gave me during my illness.

The prefects were announced one by one. Each person would be called up to stand in front of the current prefect on the stage. The current leadership team stood on a higher step, while we stood below them. That's how the pinning of the badge would take place. Slowly, one by one, they called the names of each of my classmates who had also been elected. I eagerly waited for my name to be called but it wasn't. Normally this wouldn't be a good thing, but in this situation it was great. This meant I was either going to be a school or vice-captain. I was ecstatic!

'The 2015 vice-captain and captains are....'
'Angus Cunningham, School Captain.'

Yes, that's correct; I became the captain of my primary school, Burraneer Bay Public School. It has a nice ring to it, doesn't it!

I couldn't believe it – my name had just been called. I'd been elected school captain. For a second, everything went still. Then the applause hit me, and it was like a wave crashing over my chest. At that moment, it felt like the best day of my life. I was bursting with happiness; every part of me wanted to jump up and down, scream or hug someone. But I was standing in front of the entire school, all eyes on me. So I smiled, stood tall and tried to play it cool – like I wasn't about to explode with excitement inside. It was surreal, like a dream you don't want to wake up from.

I had to then walk over to my mate Jai, who was to pin the badge on me. As my peers had all done before, it was a pretty straightforward process: The old team just put the badge on, and you got a photo. However, funny story: My mate Jai couldn't get the pin in to put the badge on me. Yep, I kid you not, here we were in front of the whole school, and Jai was fiddling around with the school captain badge. Not even joking, I think I got stabbed about four or five times with the pin as he struggled to get the damn thing in. Poor bloke, he was so embarrassed, especially when one of the teachers had to come and see if he needed assistance. He eventually got it on, and let me tell you, the badge was not put on straight at all. Such a great story though, and every time I see Jai, I still love to bring it up.

The Calm Before the Storm

With the school year wrapping up, I was beyond excited for 2015. I could already tell it was going to be my best year yet. I had a solid group of friends, I was doing well in sports and school, and I'd just been named school captain. Year 6 was ahead of me, and I was ready to take it on like never before. Everything felt like it was lining up perfectly, and I couldn't wait to see what the year had in store. I was ready for it!

Each year just before Christmas, we go to Moss Vale to spend it with Mum's side of the family. I always love going there, especially for holidays or birthdays, as Grandma loves to cook up a gigantic feast. She is Italian, so you know the stereotype: my Grandma Fran is the quintessential Italian grandmother. Perfect place to be for a young boy trying to put some weight back on! You have lunch, and you stuff your face, forgetting about dessert. I deadset think that you gain around a kilogram that day at Grandma's, and let me tell you from experience, it is so worth it. (Love you, Grandma).

It was delightful to be around the whole family as well, for a good reason. We'd all had a great year, and it was so good to be gathered together. That's why I love Christmas time so much: getting to see family that you don't usually see, everyone is happy and there is no school or work. Particularly, the weather is consistently scorching hot, making it the ideal time of year to visit the beach.

The six-week holidays were the best. You'd spend your days skating with friends, the sun on your back, and not having to worry about anything else. There's something about being a kid and just cruising around with your mates, laughing until your stomach hurts, and feeling like time is just entirely yours. Those were some of the best memories of my young life. I was able to enjoy these holidays a great deal, compared to last year, when I was still dealing with the clexane and the aftermath of the treatment. I was back to being a crazy kid and hanging out with my friends non-stop.

Every year, I always looked forward to heading to Narooma at the start of January. It's like paradise on earth – my deadset favourite place. Even to this day, we still make sure that we all get there, although it gets a lot harder the older we get! We get to see all of our cousins and family, and the whole vibe is just pure rest and relaxation. The ocean, the landscape, everything about it feels like a reset button for the year ahead. Nothing compares to it. There are really nice surfing beaches, great fishing spots, and Tilba Tilba. Every time we went to Narooma, we couldn't skip out on the Tilba Tilba visit.

There was a lolly shop that we went to, and after checking out all the other stores and markets, Mum and Dad would give us some money to go and pick out some lollies. The Tilba lolly store has just about every lolly you can think of. There were Gobstoppers the size of tennis balls, the world's sourest lollies – you name it, Tilba had it. I always opted for the Tilba gumballs; I still get them to this day. The nostalgia is now the best part as I have definitely lost my sweet tooth! Dad and I also had to get fudge from Tilba Dairy, where they sold an assortment of amazing cheeses, fresh salami and the best cream you will ever eat.

Our South Coast adventure usually signified the end of the school holidays, as we typically got home just before school was back. Except this time was different. After Narooma, we actually went to Japan for a few weeks. I know, right? We hadn't vacationed enough, had we? Japan was beautiful. We went to Hakuba and snowboarded and skied for a week, then went to visit family friends in Tokyo. Japan is one of my favourite places on earth; the people are lovely, the food is amazing and the landscape is breathtaking. I think this is where my sushi addiction started, especially sashimi. Japanese is easily one of the best cuisines.

Japan was also actually where I had my first proper nosebleed. I remember it like it was yesterday; my brothers and I were having a snowball fight (what could go wrong). Henry and I were going back and forth until he hit me square in the nose. As soon as the 'snowball' hit me, I realised that this was different from the rest. It was, in fact, an ice ball. So yes, you could imagine that my nose did not appreciate it at all. Isn't it funny the things that you remember as a kid? Mine is how my nose bled in Japan. Of course, I remember a lot more, but one of the highlights was my nose bleeding.

Anyway, this was my final holiday before a big school year was to start off, and I was ready. I was so lucky to have parents like mine and the opportunity to travel and holiday that year. I just want to thank them again for all the opportunities that they provided us. Not only that, but I just hope that they are proud of me; that's why I do what I do, to show support for what they have done for all of us boys.

The Second Diagnosis

On one of my last few nights at Narooma, I was hanging out with my cousin Hilton, who happened to be taking photos, and I hopped in one. This photo was just a normal picture of my face, with no significance whatsoever, but it wasn't until you had a closer look that you realised the alarming nature of the picture. No one noticed it until later. In that innocent photo taken in Narooma earlier in the year, you could see a swelling on my neck from a certain angle, which resembled small golf balls.

It wasn't large enough to notice in person, but you could tell from the picture that something was off. We had almost forgotten about it since I hadn't been sick in so long, so we wouldn't bother looking for minor details. Maybe if we had spotted the swelling on my neck at the time, we could have gotten on top of things earlier; maybe it would've made that year more bearable; maybe we could've avoided treatment…

These are things we will never know, and at the time we had no idea our lives once again would change forever, with repercussions that will be felt by my family and me for the rest of our lives.

This is where my second diagnosis starts. I was older, being eleven, and more knowledgeable, so I knew how serious the situation was, and this is when my mental health began to decline. For the first time in my life, I struggled greatly to stay optimistic and see the bright side of things; at times, I felt as though I had lost myself.

It was early February 2015 and the school year started off just like any other year, but there were a few giant differences. Finally, as Year 6 students, we were all excited to be the big kids at school. I was enjoying my role of being school captain, and I wore the badge proudly to school every day. And to make things even better, my class was going to be awesome! Lots of my friends were in it, and we had Mrs Cooper, who was an excellent teacher. This year had all the ingredients to be one of the best years so far.

We had a check-up with my oncologist Toby booked for late March; it was going to be a quick check-up and kind of just a recap. I was almost excited to see Toby as by this point I'd had such a great summer, topped off with snowboarding in Japan. I had so much to tell him. Usually Mum or Dad would take me in turns to these appointments. It was usually tit-for-tat; Mum would take me once, then Dad would the time after. It was coming up soon, but little did we know, one fateful night, that appointment would end up coming a few weeks sooner than anticipated.

It was late February and one night I was in my room getting ready for bed. I should probably mention that I have this habit of feeling the lymph nodes in my neck. It started after I got sick some time ago, and I continue to do it, even as I'm writing this. It's almost become like a nervous tick, sort of PTSD thing, I think. I frequently check to see if my body parts are swollen or abnormal. I witnessed everyone do it while they were investigating me, so I was familiar enough with the process to do it by myself. Anyway, as you can probably tell, I had been distracted during most of my summer holidays, which was a good thing. But I hadn't felt my neck in a while. So on this particular night, a few days before Darcy's seventh birthday, I went back to my old routine of just feeling the lymph nodes in my neck.

To my shock, it was entirely different from the other times I had done it. The right side of my neck felt as solid as concrete. When I probed it with my fingers, the lymph nodes were so swollen that they felt like a cluster of grapes pushing against my skin, their individual shapes lost in the alarming mass. Grapes are honestly even an understatement; they were like golf balls. I continually repeated the process. I think I was hoping that if I did it enough times, it would change the outcome, but of course, it didn't. I froze. A million thoughts ran through my head. *How? Everything had been so good. This doesn't make sense.*

After what seemed like an eternity, I finally came back to the present, and that's when I got up and ran into Mum and Dad's room to show them what I had discovered.

Mum and Dad, bless them, calmed me down and told me that everything was going to be okay. I was in a state of extreme distress, my mind racing frantically. This was meant to be my year; this couldn't be true. Dad had a feel of my neck and agreed that the nodes were definitely inflamed, but he reassured me that it could be a million other things. Especially since my last clear PET scan was over a year ago at this point. This helped me to calm down a bit, and I went back to bed. I was accompanied by both Mum and Dad in my bedroom this time, with hugs and reassurance. They had a good way of making sure that I would relax and not be scared. They still do, always making sure I am alright.

Despite my parents' reassurance, I didn't get much sleep that night, but I relied on their assurance that everything would be fine. My mum, however, had already booked the next available appointment for me to see Toby. I admire my parents and their strength; they were able to calm me down, even though they were probably freaking out more than I was in that situation.

I went to school the next day, and I remember telling a few of my close mates what I had discovered. Although we were all eleven years old at the time, all the boys understood the severity of the situation. Even more than myself, to be bluntly honest, as their parents had filled them in on the circumstances when I was sick the first time, and luckily I had been a bit sheltered. We all remained hopeful, and the boys did a wonderful job in ensuring that I didn't think about it too much. I found myself getting distracted and unable to think straight. My mind was flooded with questions and thoughts. Usually I was really engaged in class, but now I found myself distant and not present. This could not be happening again; this was meant to be my year.

My parents were troopers. They didn't let me know about any anxieties they may have been feeling but just kept reassuring me everything was going to be okay. What was okay, though? I was fine now, but I was not sure if I would be okay later. The fear of the unknown grew heavier with each passing day, not knowing if the cancer had returned.

It was the 26th of February 2015, only about three or four days after my lumps were discovered, and we were heading back to C2North to see Toby. I was accustomed to only Mum or Dad coming with me. On this day, however, they both decided to come with me. Alarm bells went off in my head. I tried not to make a big deal of it, but the only times both Mum and Dad would come to my appointments was when they were big appointments, such as scan results, new chemos and side effects, or my first diagnosis.

Although they maintained a calm demeanour, the car ride to the hospital was silent. You could've heard a pin drop. The vibe was so off, and although we were never 'excited' for our visits, we always had the positive outcome to rely on. I was in remission, and it had been well over six months without any signs of active cancer.

We arrived at the hospital, parked in the car park as we normally did, and began our walk towards C2North. Mum and Dad were both trying to hold my hands as we made our way up to the ward. I didn't want to hold their hands, not because I didn't appreciate them, but because my palms were so sweaty. My nails had been completely chewed off; I couldn't hide my anxiety anymore as I was so nervous. I just wanted a normal school year for my final year, and the thought of missing that cut me very deep.

I wanted to just keep being a normal kid; I'd tasted it and I enjoyed it. The hardest part wasn't just the physical distance from friends and normal life, it was the way people looked at you, the pity in their eyes. All I wanted was to blend in, to be a regular kid. Cancer made that impossible; it turned me into a spectacle, an outsider. And as much as I knew it wasn't anyone's fault, that didn't make the isolation any easier. This was what was causing my anxiety, which, funnily enough, I think that was the last thing on Mum and Dad's minds. They just wanted a healthy kid.

Once again, we were back in that all-too-familiar C2North waiting room. Except this time, I felt as though I was a lamb to the slaughter. We still hadn't seen Toby, so we couldn't be 100 per cent sure of the results, but I just had a feeling. I didn't tell Mum and Dad that or anyone, but within myself I knew that it was not good. You know how sometimes you get that feeling inside that something is off? Well, that's how I felt.

I couldn't help but pan around again while we were waiting. I experienced a sinking sensation, as though I was gazing into a mirror that reflected both my past and my imminent future. It was extremely overwhelming.

Finally, after what felt like a lifetime of waiting, Toby came to take us into the consultation room. He greeted me with his normal 'Hey Maestro', which helped to put my mind at ease a little bit. As I have mentioned earlier, Toby doesn't like to mess around at all. He got straight into the clinical observations, with many questions about how I was feeling. You know, the worst part was that everything was completely fine. I was eating well, putting on a healthy amount of weight, and fit; I was just a normal eleven-year-old kid. Everything was perfectly normal. Until he got to my neck.

He examined my neck and then proceeded to feel the lymph nodes. As Toby had a great poker face, his expression didn't really change, but his response to the nodes said everything, really. He wanted me to get an immediate PET scan, as he was fearful that the cancer had come back. Toby assured us that he didn't intend to scare us, but he was straightforward with the information. In a way, I preferred it like this – no awkward small talk, no beating around the bush. Just straight to the point, clear and honest.

He explained the steps that would take place if the PET scan didn't back clear, and how if what he thought was correct, this would be a much more complicated treatment process, which may include radiotherapy and worse. I remember hearing all this, but once again my mind was back in that dark place. My heart was racing so fast I felt as though it would beat out of my chest. My hands were all clammy, and I couldn't sit still as the nerves were too much. I just wanted to scream and wake up from this nightmare, but it was all too much. I mentally crawled back into my shell. I was so focused on the interior noise that I didn't notice what Toby and my parents were saying.

I looked over for the first time at my parents to see their reactions, and I wish I hadn't; the horror on their faces, it looked like they had seen a ghost. I felt (and still do feel) horrible as I have never seen so much angst, confusion and fear all mixed up in one. They didn't deserve this, so I felt guilty. They'd done nothing but love and care for me, and once again they were caught up in this crap. For the first time in my life, I felt terrible for being their kid. I just wanted them to be happy, like they were when we were in the Northern Territory or in Japan, not looking how they did at this moment in time. The fear of the unknown was etched on their faces. Toby finished talking and asked his famous line, 'Questions?' I don't remember my answer to this question; I don't even know if I spoke another word for the rest of the day. Although nothing was confirmed, and we had to wait for the PET scan results, as I mentioned earlier… I knew.

I was booked in to get a PET scan a few days after the initial appointment. Those days were just a complete blur as I couldn't even think straight. I had way too much on my mind, and I was struggling a lot with the situation that was unfolding. The days were passing quickly, and everything appeared to be beyond my control. I felt kind of helpless and lost. The days of me being sick had been a distant memory, and now they weren't. It had become my reality again in such a short period of time. I had been on holiday just a month before, and now I found myself in a hospital undergoing scans for cancer. It was a giant burden on me; I could only imagine how my parents felt. Here I was, sitting in another PET scan machine. I had vowed to myself that I would never end up in one of these again, but look at me now.

The next day's results confirmed my fears. The cancer had returned with a vengeance, forming masses on both sides of my neck and spreading to my stomach. While cancer recurrences aren't typically staged, this aggressive return would have been classified as stage III, a stark reminder of its progression beyond the initial diagnosis in my neck. However, I remained asymptomatic, which was a positive sign, indicating that I was still in stage A. We were all extremely distraught and anxious. This was a horrible time in our lives, and I wouldn't wish it on my worst enemy.

Not as Straightforward

For the first time in almost two years, we saw Toby twice in one week. He wanted to explain the process to us and let us know what we were about to endure. He then gave us the rundown, as he liked to do (very organised man, I'll give him that).

I was going to go have another lymph node biopsy to take a few of them out for further testing. This was going to be done on the 5th of March 2015. With the prospect of more intensive treatment looming, I was scheduled to have a central line inserted. Unlike the portacath, this was a more permanent fixture: a thin, flexible tube threaded through a vein in my chest and leading directly to a larger vein near my heart. It would serve as a highway for chemotherapy, medications and nutrition, and a route for frequent blood draws. It was like two cords hanging out of my chest, and let me tell you, it was a huge pain in the arse.

Furthermore, it had to be cleaned regularly to make sure of no infection, and you couldn't get it wet. Yes, that is correct; this was going to make showering extremely difficult as it was placed in the middle of my chest. Toby believed that the best plan was to do a brentuximab and augmented ICE trial, followed by an autologous stem cell transplant after achieving a clear PET scan. Before anyone asks, yes, ICE was one of the treatments I was to have. No, it is not what you're thinking of as the drug ice; it is an abbreviation for a bunch of nasty chemotherapies. However, I must admit that I raised an eyebrow when I learned I was receiving ice. I mean, you would too, wouldn't you?

Does anyone remember my dear old friend, the clexane needles that I had to have due to my blood clot? Since I was now at risk of getting blood clots due to a foreign object staying in my vein for an extended period, I needed to have the injections again. This was so disheartening, as the needles suck, as I mentioned earlier, and would again make physical activity impossible to do as my blood would be considerably thinner, which makes bleeding way easier. You can't bleed or have any bumps or bruises as blood that doesn't clot can be life-threatening. Imagine how stoked I was to find out this, just adding insult to injury.

This regimen was the set plan, and if everything went smoothly, it was what was going to happen. Toby had a plan in place, and we were determined to adhere to it strictly, as he had gained our complete trust. This time, however, Toby's usual optimism was tempered. The diagnosis wasn't as straightforward and the path to treatment wasn't as clear. His words, while still kind, lacked the same reassurance we'd come to expect. He shared a haunting statistic with my parents, a fact I didn't fully understand until much later in my life. I am grateful that this information never reached me, as it would have profoundly shaken me if it hadn't already.

So to put it bluntly, pretty much I had a 50/50 chance. Yes, that is correct, a coin flip. Due to the diagnosis being a reoccurrence, the cancer would've adapted and been more resistant to chemotherapy and other treatments. The odds were stark: a fifty per cent chance of the cancer returning. The severe implications were clear, even if unspoken. This wasn't just a setback for me; it was a life-threatening reality. The fight ahead was daunting, but all I knew was to keep my head up and continue moving forward. I mean, what else can you do? I am so grateful that Mum and Dad didn't let me know the statistics that were stacked against me. Even though I found out much later how horrific it actually was, I didn't need to know it at all as it wouldn't have helped my situation.

Even without knowing this statistic, the recurring cancer news really rocked me. My optimism and positive mindset, which I usually had throughout my life, had faded a bit at the start of my second diagnosis. I found myself thinking about all the negatives. I was so eager for a great year and felt as if this had all been stripped away from me. Toby couldn't really give us a straight answer with treatment completion time, as everything was kind of up in the air. I just wasn't ready to go through everything all again. Especially when I was now that bit older and understood what situation we were in at the time and how dire it really was.

My mates assured me, though, that they were going to stick by my side the whole step of the way. I was also confident in them because they would come over and hang out when I was sick. This really shows what type of friends I had (and still have); no matter how much of a couch potato I was, the usual active and busy boys would take it down a notch and relax with me, even if it just meant watching a movie or playing PlayStation. This meant a lot to me, and it made me feel reassured. It helped me get over my devastation of missing out on my cricket season. We had made the grand final at the time, but I wasn't able to play due to the diagnosis. Despite not playing, the coach let me manage the boys, and I still received an award at the end. Not one of the boys on my team or even the others treated me any different; everyone just made me feel welcome. This is a testament to the people in my community, and for them, I will always be grateful.

All my friends back at school were still shocked though. I will never forget the day I told everyone that my illness had returned. I was scared and confused, but I felt as though it was necessary, as they had always had my back and I couldn't exclude them from this. We were just kids, and suddenly we were facing something way bigger than us. The news didn't just shock them – it shattered the sense of normal we all took for granted.

My treatment plan with brentuximab was approved shortly after my surgery. The protocol followed a 28-day cycle, during which I received 1.2 mg/kg of the chemotherapy drug brentuximab vedotin through my central line on days 1, 8 and 15. This cycle was scheduled to repeat once more, identical to the first, which meant I would have two cycles all up. The good thing about this chemo was that it was a new drug that had come out, and it was a targeted therapy. It was apparently meant to have little to no side effects. I was very happy about that, as it meant that it was going to delay my hair from falling out, and I was able to miss less school so I could still fulfil my school captain's role. This was also good for my mental health, as I wasn't going to feel violently ill as you do with most chemotherapies. So I was happy that it was kind of an ease into the new treatment process. Toby also wanted PET scans done after the end of both cycles to monitor the regression of the cancer.

My first brentuximab was to be done in late March 2015 as an outpatient through C2North. As I said earlier, this treatment was meant to have fewer side effects so I could come in and get it done and leave. This was also only a 30-minute infusion, which, compared to other chemos, was a quick and easy process. I also wouldn't lose my appetite, so for me, this wasn't too bad. My diet wasn't the best, but we just had to try to get me to eat as much as possible. Lots of fried foods, and burgers. Plus, with the central line, I didn't have to get needles anymore like I did with the portacath. After the first initial shock of my re-diagnosis, I noticed that I was able to bring myself back to the positive mindset that I was always known for having. This was due to the way this cycle was to be completed: being an outpatient and going home after treatment was perfect for me. I literally remember only having tiredness as a side effect of brentuximab, which was fine as it usually passed after the initial transfusion day.

Before I even realised it, I had finished my first chemo treatment and was ready to head home. *I can do this*, I thought to myself. This brentuximab stuff wasn't bad at all; I was actually very happy with how the process was going. I would only miss one day of school for the infusion as I was a little worn out afterwards, but I would be at school completely fine the next day, running around and continuing to be a crazy kid. It allowed me to feel as though I was normal, and as I was so used to chemotherapies making me feel extremely unwell, this was a nice change. At this point, I was thrilled with brentuximab compared to other drugs I had previously taken. This was by far the winner, and it helped to keep my mind at ease. Unfortunately, this would be very short-lived; little did I know what was going to happen on Day 15 of my first cycle. It changed my life forever, with repercussions I still feel to this day.

It was early April 2015, and just like I said before, I was having my third dose of brentuximab on Day 15. I was lying on my hospital bed, speaking with a friend on the phone. We were just chatting, and as he was away on a holiday, we had a lot to talk about. He was keeping me company while the chemo was being pumped through my drip. I was just laughing and having a good time when all of a sudden I felt this weird itch in my throat. It was extremely odd, but I didn't think anything of it. However, almost immediately following the itch, I noticed that I was struggling to get my words out to my mate. I felt as though someone was squeezing my throat, and it was terrifying; it was becoming harder and harder to breathe. I didn't want to scare my friend, though, so I just quickly said, 'I've got to go,' and hung up. I threw my phone down, and that is when I started to realise the dire situation.

After the phone call finished, I was now in a full state of panic as my breaths became shorter and shorter; it had now become a fight to get some oxygen in. My chest was tight, my heart racing and I felt as though my face was on fire. I yelled out to Mum, who was next to me, 'I CAN'T BREATHE.' In an instant, Mum had called the nurses over and came over to try and assist me in any way that she could.

This was one of the most terrifying experiences of my life. Those few seconds before the nurses rushed into the room, I was there gasping for air. The tears were flooding down my face, and I thought that this was going to be the end of the road. I went from being relaxed one minute to being unable to breathe the next. It was horrifying.

Luckily, the nurses got to me quickly and put an oxygen mask on me while simultaneously stopping the brentuximab. This slowly seemed to ease the symptoms, which was a good thing. I had just experienced one of the severe side effects of the so-called 'miracle drug' I once praised before that fateful day. This was really difficult for me to comprehend, as it wasn't making me sick, and apart from a little tiredness, I was able to be a normal kid. Then all of a sudden, I was in this situation, being unable to breathe.

Shortness of breath and breathing difficulties were two severe side effects that rarely happened as a result of having brentuximab, and somehow I drew the short straw and experienced them both. I might just add that at the time I may have been one of the unluckiest people. After I finished treatment, I got a blood clot and a recurrence; luckily, I wasn't buying any lottery tickets. They were not sure why it happened or if it was going to happen again, so they sat with me and monitored me for about an hour.

After what felt like an eternity, I was cleared to continue having the brentuximab, but at a much, much slower rate. It usually took about thirty minutes to go all the way through the drip, but they slowed it down to where it would be about a two-hour process. I was nervous the whole time the drug was in the IV, but we got through it in the end. Both Mum and I were exhausted by the end of the day, as it had been extremely stressful and draining, and I was ready to take on a new day and leave this one behind.

So I woke up the next morning, after having an awful sleep, as I kept on getting that same feeling that I'd had the day before. For the first time in my life, I felt extremely on edge and experienced heightened anxiety.

That morning, I kept on reliving the traumatic experience of the day before, and I felt that I couldn't eat food and that I kept on having that weird itch in my throat. This was causing me a great amount of distress, and I remember being very emotional as I was scared about everything happening again. Mum was very worried about me, and she took me back into the hospital to get checked out, as I was in so much fear. Everything from eating to just lying around had become a massive struggle, as I kept on feeling that same feeling, which would in time freak me out.

The hospital checked me out, and everything was fine. They told me that all my vitals were good; it was just that I was having panic attack episodes as a result of the trauma I'd experienced the day prior. This was the start of my anxiety and post-traumatic stress disorder (PTSD) that would make these next eighteen months extremely difficult, as it caused me a great amount of stress. This would end up making the entire process become even more challenging than it already was. I became very fearful of dying, experiencing frequent panic attacks.

For the majority of the treatment process as well, I believed that I had a lump in my throat that would stop me from being able to breathe, which made eating and drinking hard. I couldn't stop thinking about that little boy from 2013 – the one I saw wheeled away to ICU. So small, so fragile, swallowed by machines and tubes. That image haunted me. No matter how hard I tried to shake it, a part of me kept believing that was going to be me. I'd lie in bed, staring at the ceiling, picturing myself in his place – hooked up, fading, disappearing. It was like I'd glimpsed a version of my future I couldn't unsee.

Managing Anxiety

At the time, we didn't realise how massive that fateful day was going to be, but as I mentioned earlier, the effects of that day I still feel today with my anxiety and PTSD from the situation. The thing is though, most people wouldn't even know as I try to hide it. Only the people really close to me know how severe my anxiety is and can get.

So that was my first real introduction to anxiety and PTSD, which happened when I was eleven, just shy of twelve years old. My birthday was April 22, and for the first time, I was going to have cancer. This made parties and everything else extremely difficult, as we needed to watch for bugs and any other nasty things that go around, as it would have made me very unwell. But having the beautiful family that I did, Mum and Dad didn't want me to miss out.

So for my twelfth birthday, my parents hired out a room in the movie theatre for all my friends and family. I was so excited, and I even had a few of my close mates able to stay the night after. This was one positive of the brentuximab: my immunity was still relatively good, so I could enjoy a fun night out with my friends and feel included. The movie idea was also a good one, as it was nice and relaxing, and as I had two cords coming out of my chest with the central line, I could also participate with no other worries about bumping them or getting them wet.

I can't remember if I mentioned it or not, but yeah, you can't get the central line wet, so it was a lot of bathing with a sponge for the unforeseen future. The classic sponge baths, how fun! To be honest, though, I used the time to have a little relaxation and take my mind off the recent events that had occurred, which was much needed.

After the reaction to brentuximab, it made the rest of the cycles a lot different. As I mentioned earlier, if I wasn't feeling worn out after the treatments, I could usually make it to school after or the next day. Now, they would make the IVs go slower and monitor for any severe symptoms like the one I'd had. I always felt my anxiety levels rise on treatment days, and during chemo sessions, I struggled with a sensation of shortness of breath. The symptoms felt so real, but they were all in my head. I found myself missing more and more school, which was the polar opposite of what was originally anticipated with the brentuximab, as it would just cause me extreme amounts of stress.

I even found eating and taking medications a massive struggle, as anything that could cause me to 'stop breathing' in my mind would cause a panic attack. This was a really hard time for me; fighting cancer is already hard enough in itself, and then having panic attacks and anxiety all the time on top of it made it dreadful. Any weird feeling would set off a panic attack, and I would freak out. My parents and family were fantastic to me at the time, as I couldn't really talk to my mates about it as no one really understood because we were so young. I felt bad for my family as I could see them struggling to see me in such fear each time I had the treatments. They just wanted to help in any way they could, but it would just freak me out.

The brentuximab cycles couldn't have finished any quicker. After fifty-six days and two cycles of the drug, I had finally completed the first part of my treatment. On a positive note, though, it was noticeable that my neck had definitely shrunk in size, which was a very good sign. Especially considering the fact that it was a newer treatment, so any type of success was good. Following the protocol, I was to have a PET and CT scan within a week of finishing the treatment to check out how the cancer was going and to see how much it had regressed. We were hopeful that it was going to be some positive news.

Quick intermission: Apologies for the negative vibes during this last bit of the book. I just want to keep it real with how I was feeling at the time. Don't worry, I wasn't a neg the whole time; it was just a dark peri-

od. Bear with me as the Angus we all know and love will be back soon. Much love.

We were correct! The news was awesome. The brentuximab had actually done its job quite well. There was an obvious reduction of the mass on both sides of my neck, and it was estimated to be about a thirty per cent reduction. My stomach lymph nodes were still visible, and not much had changed, but it was a small win nonetheless. As Toby wasn't quite sure how effective the treatment was going to be, it was also a relief to know that the chemo was killing the cancer cells. It took our breath away (mine quite literally!).

The news was great, but we still had a long way to go. The support we were receiving at this time as well was amazing. The community was organising dinners for my family to take the stress off. Quick shoutout to Suzanne for orchestrating this; we are so thankful to you and everyone for donating their dinners to us.

So now we were up to the next step in my fight, the ICE protocol. This chemotherapy protocol is a combination treatment that is commonly used for relapsed Hodgkin lymphoma. There are three drugs: ifosfamide, cytarabine and etoposide. These drugs work together to prevent cancer cells from growing and dividing. It is used as a thing called salvage therapy, which pretty much is for patients whose cancer has not responded well to treatment. This is a highly aggressive cancer regimen, accompanied by a never-ending list of severe side effects. Some of the most common ones are nausea, hair loss, fatigue and low blood cell counts. When reading up on it, I also found that organ toxicity sometimes occurs, which is probably why I was in the hospital while receiving this treatment, as it is completely different from brentuximab.

Toby told us I'd be very ill and lose all my hair during this treatment phase. Sidenote, when Toby tells you something is definitely certain, you know it's going to happen, so I knew my luscious locks days were once again numbered. I would also have to isolate myself from people as well whenever I was home, as my immune system was going to be compromised. This made seeing mates difficult, but if they were healthy, it was usually okay. I had actually avoided any unwanted hospital overnights up until this point, which was good. So annoying, as I had so much good to say about brentuximab, but after that reaction, let's just say I can't exactly give it a glowing review anymore!

My parents dreaded this next phase of the chemotherapy; however, I wasn't as caught up in it all. I was taking the reduction as a win, and I kind of didn't look too much into the other stuff. Mum, Dad and Toby had many meetings and phone calls without me present during this time, which was completely fine with me. It felt like the old saying, 'What you don't know won't hurt you,' which couldn't have been more correct in this situation. I believe we gained valuable insights from the list of side effects associated with brentuximab. Although the list was short, there were certain cases where a person who had previously eaten contaminated meat during the mad cow disease epidemic had the virus dormant in their body, but it flared back up after treatment, and they ended up getting the disease. For the next week after I learned that, I stayed up researching and stressing about mad cow disease and that I might have it. So that was one of the last side effect meetings I ever sat in. My perspective on health was all over the place; any time I had any sickness, I immediately thought the worst, which just caused more anxiety. It was a rough cycle, to say the least.

It was May the 16th and the plan was set: I was going to be hospitalised during the start of the ICE cycle, which included four days straight of chemotherapy. This was going to be a week from hell; I was going to be very, very ill at the conclusion of the cycle, so it was important that I looked after myself. I was going to be admitted on the 17th, so as Mum and Dad were rushing around and getting me organised for my 'holiday', I had a plan. Around this time, soccer – or football for my Europeans – was another sport I enjoyed participating in and also playing on my PlayStation. Ronaldo was my favourite player, so what better way to show this than to get his haircut? This was very unlike me, as I always had a blonde fringe or long hair, but his hair at the time was short, with the back and sides, and gelled to the side. The haircut didn't suit me at all, but I knew my hair was not leaving the hospital with me, so I decided the best time to try it was now.

The night before the hospital, I was having two of my best mates over, Jarvis and Vaughan. These boys were so good to me and always hung out with me no matter what situation I was in. They would sit with me when I couldn't do much or join me in skateboarding (even if they weren't very good at it) or whatever I wanted to try. They were, and still are, incredible humans. Furthermore, they were to stay the night as a kind of little send-off for me, as the next few weeks/months were going to be really hard with starting my intense chemotherapy regime. The CALM before the STORM, should I say. Well, my mum, being the best, made my favourite dinner for me: roast pork. It was delicious and the perfect meal to have. However, little did we know what was going to happen that night. Side note: someone up there somewhere has to be looking at my life and just taking the piss, honestly. I hope they are having a laugh at my expense; I am whilst reading this as you cannot make this up.

So let me set the scene. Usually with sleepovers, you try to stay awake until the latest, but I needed a good rest, and the boys respected that. By good rest, we still stayed up until like midnight but not the usual all-nighter. Actually, I forgot to mention the delicious roast pork was cooked on the BBQ. We didn't realise we forgot to turn it off. I'm sure you can figure out where this is going.

At around two a.m., I forgot which brother, but one of them saw a light coming from downstairs. This was odd, they thought, but instead of going to investigate it, they didn't think too much of it. They didn't realise, nor did anyone else in the family, that the unturned-off BBQ had caught fire and spread to our fence. No word of a lie, our house was on fire. May I add that this was the night before I was set to go into the hospital and have chemo? My poor parents couldn't catch a break, am I right? My mum woke us up and yelled at us to leave the house immediately.

Being kids, we had to quickly run up the stairs to see what was going on, which is when I witnessed something no kid should ever have to see. My dad was in boxer shorts with a hose trying to fight this fire. It is hilarious looking back, but at the time, it was a sight. The fire was huge though; it had spread to our fence and a bit onto our house. Mum grabbed us and raced us out the front. The firefighters got to our house in an instant, which was a giant relief. Talk about a sleepover, am I right? The whole street was on the road, looking at the commotion that had gone on. The smoke was immense, completely smothering the sky.

Luckily, we were all fine, and the house only suffered minor damage. The firefighters contained the blaze quickly, sparing us from anything worse. In the end, some positives came out of the chaos: our BBQ area had to be renovated, and now it looks better than ever. Oh, and for everyone wondering, no, Dad's boxers didn't make it. They were beyond saving and had to be tossed out. What a night to remember! Reflecting on it, how crazy was the timing? What a way to send me off for my treatment.

After all the debacle from last night, it was time to start the ICE cycle. On May 17th my Cristiano Ronaldo haircut and I were in the car on the way to the hospital. Despite having experienced this battle before, I couldn't help but feel nervous. But I was also excited about the up-and-coming State of Origin between the NSW Blues and the QLD Maroons. This was always one of my favourite times of the year, as I am sure you can remember what happened the year prior. Unfortunately, I wasn't going to strip off naked and run around if the Blues won this year, though. I was still, however, not going to miss watching the first game on the 27th of May for anything.

The ICE Cycle

If I had a dollar for every time someone mentioned the severity of the ICE protocol, I wouldn't be a millionaire, but I'd be pretty darn close. We were constantly getting briefed about what would happen and the side effects. The possibility of a feeding tube was also something that they were considering, as I wouldn't be able to eat as I would be extremely ill, either vomiting or sleeping for large amounts of time. The feeding tube was my arch nemesis, to put it simply. Up until this far in my cancer journey, I hadn't had the pleasure of engaging with it yet, but the look of the tube was frightening. It gives me goosebumps writing this; honestly, they are terrible.

The tube itself is very helpful when you can't eat, but getting it set is horrendous. Pretty much, to set up a nasogastric feeding tube, it involves inserting a long pipe up your nose, and you have to keep swallowing the whole time to make sure it enters your stomach and not your lungs accidentally.

Throughout the process, you must resist the urge to sneeze, and your eyes are filled with tears. I can't even put into words how terrible it is. Anyway, with that thought looming on my mind, I was going to try and eat as much food as possible. I hadn't even had a feeding tube yet; just the sight of it sent shivers down my spine.

The day had arrived for the start of the chemotherapy cycle. I don't know if you have noticed, but I am not saying I was ready because I wasn't. The anxiety I was feeling was tremendous, and I wasn't prepared in any way for the mountain I was about to climb. I had become so accustomed to the relatively mild side effects of the previous treatment that I had almost forgotten how to cope with the overwhelming side effects of chemotherapy. Especially when being told it would be the strongest I'd ever had before.

It was very surreal when the all-too-familiar sight of the nurses appeared dressed head to toe in gowns, holding bags wrapped in duct tape. You could cut the tension in the air with a knife. I remember this being the exact moment everything truly hit me. My throat felt as if it was closing up, and my heart was racing a thousand beats a minute. My anxiety was consuming me completely. I didn't want to tell my mum, who was with me, because they had already been through so much. At just twelve years old, I was sitting there getting ready for my body to be filled with these toxins, which are meant to kill you, but just as much, they were meant to assist you in your fight for survival.

This 'medicine', however, brings pain and exhaustion, but also hope that somewhere in the suffering, healing was happening. I liked to look at the treatment as fighting fire with fire. I don't know why, but it made me feel braver, like a warrior. I remember the first lot of chemo coming through as a weird, reddish colour. This was very unsettling, to be honest. Let's just say it did not look like it should be going into a human body. The strange colour of the chemo – that reddish hue – has stayed with me. It was hard to shake the feeling that something so unnatural should never be inside your body. But there was a weird sort of reassurance in knowing that it was doing its job, even if it felt more like a poison than medicine. I couldn't help but wonder if this was the price I had to pay for survival, the ultimate test of endurance. Despite the pain and the toll it took on my body, there was always that sliver of hope, that to get out of it, you had to go through it.

A few days and several more chemo sessions with strange, unsettling colours had passed; it was now the 27th of May. The side effects had appeared, and my god, had they come on strong. I was extremely nauseous and unwell. I was fragile, with nonstop fluids coming out of both ends. My usual chatty self was quiet and disengaged. I struggled to eat, and whatever I managed to consume wouldn't stay down. I was taking anti-nausea medication such as ondansetron like they were tic tacs, and still, nothing was helping with the nausea. I would sleep for the majority of the day, and when I wasn't asleep, I was either vomiting or in pain. I was having a hard time, but tonight's State of Origin helped boost my spirits a little.

My weight had dropped severely, and my kidney function was noticeably down, which was a little bit of a concern for the doctors, so they had to manage that closely. On a more positive note, though, my Year 6 jersey was dropped off at the hospital that day, which was a giant moment for me. I had waited all my life for this jersey, and to finally have it was great. It made me look forward to the future. I could already see my mates and me laughing and playing back at school in our jerseys; it was going to be so fun. The jersey was such a minuscule item to most my age, but for me, it represented so much more, and it helped me to keep on pushing on and continue to see the light at the end of the tunnel.

Even in times like this, it is so easy to get bogged down and focus on the negatives, but reflecting on one good thing can help change your mindset completely. I'm grateful for the time I got to spend with my parents, and even though most of the time I wasn't feeling great, this is when I realised how much love and support can carry you through the hardest moments. Just their presence, even if nothing was being said, made everything a little more bearable.

The Origin was a very close game, but unfortunately the Maroons snuck away with the win by one point, with the final score being 10–11. I hate to admit it, but during this time it was an all-too-familiar sight of us getting beaten by the Queenslanders. 'Our time will come,' I would always say, but for now it was not our time.

After the first cycle of ICE was completed, Toby and the nursing staff allowed me to go home for a bit before the second cycle started.

On the 28th, they sent me home, which was amazing! However, it only lasted about sixteen hours before I was back in the hospital. In my short stint at home, I had my first glimpse of myself in the mirror, and what I saw was shocking. I am going to have a crack at a descriptive sentence to try and paint the picture for you guys of how crook I was looking. My eyes were sunken deep into my face, rimmed with dark circles, and my skin had taken on a ghostly pallor, clinging to the sharp angles of my face, leaving me looking like a shadow of the person I once was. *Jeez, now that is not bad at all. Pat on the back for that sentence; I am proud of it.*

All jokes aside, but yeah, it kind of scared me, honestly. I couldn't even recognise my reflection, which is a very weird feeling. It probably was a good thing I was right back to the hospital; I definitely needed it. I should also clarify that each hospital admission is typically due to high fevers, severe nausea or an inability to eat or drink. Contrary to what you might think, I was not going there for a quick holiday, I promise!

So on the 29th of May, after a solid sixteen hours at home, I was back. This time, I had a few companions by my side, three to be exact. And I'm not talking about people, but pumps. That's right, there were that many chords going into me it wasn't even funny. I liked to think I was like Iron Man a little bit – except way less powerful and more bedridden – but it made me happy, so that's all that mattered. As I said earlier, even taking the piss out of certain situations helped me so much. A quote I lived by and still continue to do goes as follows: 'You can either laugh or you can cry,' and honestly, it's so true.

My immunity was pretty much non-existent at this point, with my kidneys still on struggle street. I needed a platelet transfusion to try and boost my immune system a little bit, as it is very, very dangerous when you have no immunity, as I'm sure you can imagine. The platelets were in this big bright-yellow bag that literally looked like the colour of corn; it was disgusting. I had to be isolated as well, as any germs from anyone else would be life-threatening. Every time a nurse checked on me, she wore a mask and gown to protect me from any potential infections. On the bright side, it was nice in the isolation room. You didn't have three other kids' pumps all going off at the same time, so it was considerably quieter. I forgot to mention I was in a new ward, which was exciting. I was now in C3West, which was a level above my usual hangout spots at C2North and C2West.

Getting food down was becoming an even greater struggle than it had been before. I managed to eat a cutlet and half an apple, though each bite felt like a victory, my stomach rebelling with every chew, as if even the simplest tasks were too much to ask. My poor mum would make or buy any food I desired and bring it to me to encourage me to eat. I felt terrible, as I could tell how much both she and Dad wanted me to eat, but I just physically couldn't. On a positive note, though, my tumours in my neck were 'appearing' to be smaller from our perspective, which meant that this nasty chemo was doing its job.

To everyone who is also wondering what it feels like to go through chemotherapy, I will try to describe it as best as possible: It is like the worst stomach bug in the world. You feel terrible with non-stop vomiting and diarrhoea (sorry, too much information, but it's the only way to describe it), and also weak, exhausted and fatigued all the time. There are days when you will pretty much just sleep the whole day, as your body is trying to fight away this cancer with the assistance of chemo. You then get run down pretty much from all the vomiting and the rest, so you get blisters and stuff in your mouth and other areas as the stuff coming out of you is toxic. So hygiene is of the utmost priority when you are going through cancer treatment. It does make it hard, though, when you have a bunch of cords hanging out of your chest, but you try and make do.

I remember once Dad thought of an idea to wrap my central line in plastic wrap and attempt to have a normal shower. This did not go well, and water ended up getting all the way through it. Everything ended up being fine, but if possible, it is best not to get the line wet, as an infected line would cause significant issues, especially when the line leads into my heart. Yeah, it wouldn't be good at all.

The love and overwhelming support my family and I were getting during this time, too, was amazing. Each night, a different family was dropping food off to our house for the boys to eat, which allowed for one less thing my parents had to worry about. Our friends and family also helped take my brothers to their sports training, tutoring and school, which helped enormously. The fight against cancer isn't won by the individual; it is won by the surrounding team. In my case, my family, friends and extended community backed me every step of the way. It demonstrated the immense power of love and support during life's most challenging struggles.

On the morning of May 31st, just a few days into my second cycle of the infamous ICE protocol, I was absentmindedly scratching my head when I noticed something alarming: a gap had formed where my hair used to be. It was as if patches were vanishing before my eyes, and that's when the realisation hit me: my hair was starting to go, and it was happening fast. Don't ask why, but I kept on literally just pulling my hair out; I was grabbing chunks of it and throwing it in the bin. I was sick of being in the hospital and not being able to see anyone, so with the frustration, I just took it out on my hair. I started the day with a head full of hair and ended it with no hair. In just a few hours, I transformed into a completely different person. It's actually quite funny when you think about it. I've heard the saying 'pulling your hair out' countless times throughout my life to describe stress or frustration, and I quite literally did it.

Stem Cell Harvest

After the chemo was finished, I was to get my stem cells harvested in preparation for my autologous stem cell transplant. Now, this was going to make the ICE protocol look like a walk in the park. An autologous stem cell transplant was the most daunting but crucial step in my fight; it is usually reserved as a back-up option when other treatments haven't done the job. The process involves collecting healthy stem cells from your blood after being pumped full of medication to boost their production. These little lifesavers are then frozen and safely stored for what's to come.

Next up was the part no one looks forward to: extremely high-dose chemotherapy for about a week straight. It's designed to obliterate cancer cells but also takes out your bone marrow's ability to produce blood cells, leaving you completely reliant on those stored stem cells. Then comes the reinfusion. Your thawed stem cells are reintroduced into your bloodstream, where they make their way back to your bone marrow and begin the hard work of rebuilding your blood and immune system.

The recovery is slow and frustrating, but those stem cells eventually do their job, offering a chance to bounce back from the intense toll of the chemo. It's far from easy, but in the battle against cancer, this procedure can be the lifeline that turns the tide. Stem cell transplants are an extremely risky process, as you have zero immunity for a substantial amount of time. You are kept in the hospital in isolation for at least a month, though there's no set time limit. You stay until your body fully accepts the stem cells. There is also a small risk that the stem cells get rejected, which creates a whole other issue. With this at the back of our minds, we knew the massive fight that we had coming up, but one thing we did know is that we weren't going to fight it alone at all. Once you are out of the hospital, you are not out of danger yet, as recovery usually takes between three to six months.

The day my stem cells were to be harvested, we ran into a problem: my blood pressure was dangerously low. It was a funny day, to be honest, as the nurses kept rushing in, alarmed by how dangerously low my blood pressure had dropped, treating it like a full-blown emergency. To their surprise, each time they ran in, I was just sitting up eating my crackers, without a care in the world. There were even talks of sending me to the ICU as that's how low it was. I thought it was all a big joke, to be honest. Between that and the dietitian, it was not one of my most pleasant days in the hospital, I'll say that much.

Ah yes, the Sydney Children's dietitian – now wasn't she my favourite person ever? Not! Look, if you're out there, I'll apologise now for ignoring you and trying to avoid you. But in my defence, trying to make a sick, not hungry kid eat by threatening them with a feeding tube wasn't exactly a recipe for friendship. She would always tell me to eat and leave it at that, but if it were really that simple, I would've done it a long time ago. I was literally skin and bones, and believe me, I loved my food (still do); I wasn't trying to be difficult.

I had to wait two more days before I could get my stem cells harvested. They were keeping me in the hospital for four days anyway, so I just had to do it two days later than anticipated. This was definitely one of the scariest and strangest days of my life, getting my stem cells harvested. I've mentioned a few times already the bunch of cords hanging out of my chest, known as a central line. Well, to harvest my stem cells (and just thinking about it still gives me shivers), they connected those cords to a large machine that filtered my blood. Yes, you read that right: they actually filtered my blood to collect the stem cells. You could actually watch litres of your blood being pulled out of your body, going through the machine, and then being pumped back in.

It still makes me feel queasy just thinking about it – so unnatural and wrong. It is understandable why this couldn't be done with low blood pressure, isn't it? This process took approximately six hours. That is all I am going to speak on that day, as it gives me the chills. The experience was unsettling for me. Anyway, after the stem cells were harvested, they managed to stabilise my low blood pressure, so they kept me in the hospital for a few more days just to monitor things. They administered platelet and blood transfusions to combat my low immunity and aid in my recovery.

Platelet infusions were very odd; as I've said, they came in bright yellow bags. I knew how helpful it was, but I couldn't stop thinking about how disgusting it looked. There was something about the thick golden liquid being pumped into my veins that made my stomach turn. Here's a quick reminder to donate blood if you can; you'll never know who needs it, and it could potentially save someone's life.

On June 5th, I finally received my release and was able to return home.

When we were leaving the hospital, Mum decided that she wanted to drive me out to Kurnell to watch the sunset with her. This was a great decision, as it was one of the most beautiful sunsets I have ever seen in my life. I can still see it now, the deep orange stretching across the horizon, and something about it calmed me. Nature is amazing, and I recommend to anyone struggling in any battles or with anything to go outside and enjoy the beauty that is around us. Even just looking at the night sky outside a hospital bed was a moment in time I'll never forget; it reminded me how grateful I was just to be alive and present. Thanks for that one, Mum; I will treasure that moment forever.

My ICE journey was now complete after countless hospital stays/visits and, honestly, one of the hardest months of my life. I looked like an entirely different person, and my spirits definitely dropped at times, but I got through it. I will always give credit to the love and support my family received as well during this hard time; we were never alone. My brothers were also looked after by a whole range of people, with a big shout-out to Grandma and Pop for coming from Southern Highlands to come and look after them. Now, we just hoped that the chemo killed the cancer as well as it almost killed me!

Unfortunately, the scan wasn't promising at all. My PET scan revealed that the chemo was effective in pretty much everything but killing my cancer. There was little to no change in the scan, with the cancer still very visible. In fact, the spread of cancer appeared to have increased. Like, come on, are you kidding me?

This was not good, with Toby not factoring this in at all. It portrayed how the cancer had adapted over time, and we were kind of running out of options, as the ICE protocol was meant to kill the majority of the cancer then I'd be ready for my transplant. We needed to regroup and allow for Toby the genius to brainstorm other options to kill this bastard of a thing. I can't lie, it was an emotional night when the results came, as what kept me pushing through the whole ICE ordeal was the fact that I believed my cancer was shrinking with this horrible treatment.

I used to tell myself, 'I can survive this, but the cancer can't.' Turns out I was entirely wrong; the cancer was surviving, and I was barely! This was a time in my treatment where things weren't looking positive, and that night my optimism faded for a bit. But these things happen, and sometimes you just have to allow yourself a few tears and a little time to process it, and then you have to pick yourself up and carry on. As much as things can set you back, life doesn't wait for anyone, and you have to keep on going.

After a brief reflection, I realised that I shouldn't take this as a loss but as a win. I survived this scary chemotherapy regime that so many people had warned me about. Granted, it took my hair and probably about ten kilograms, but it couldn't keep me down, and I would keep on smiling the whole way through. I'll tell you what it wasn't capable of taking: my eyebrows, even though I was told they wouldn't make it. So, I'm counting that as a win: Angus 1, ICE Chemo Protocol 0. Better luck next time, loser (hopefully no next time; it did suck).

Michael Ennis Visits

It was the 13th of June 2015. After every storm, there is a rainbow, and my rainbow came as a Cronulla Sharks hooker, who was arguably one of the biggest grubs in the NRL at the time. However, after meeting him, I can confirm he was one of the loveliest blokes I have ever met in my life. This was a very significant day in my cancer journey, and in my eyes pretty much sums up the goodness of my community. One of Mum's friends knew Michael well and told him how I was a die-hard Sharks fan. Out of pure kindness, he reached out to Mum and arranged a day to visit and surprise me.

What meant the most to me is that he did this in his own spare time, no media attention with cameras or anything. He just rocked up solo and spent the day with me. I do have a bone to pick, however. He beat me every time in FIFA; like, surely he could've let the cancer kid win once but no, he demolished me. He then sat down with us and had tea and lunch and filled us in on all the insights of being a professional league player. At the time, that was my dream job, so I was genuinely interested in the conversation and greatly appreciated him spending his day with us.

Shoutout as Mic Ennis is considered my greatest of all time (GOAT), and he led the Sharks to a premiership win the following year. I wish I stayed in contact with him, but that's all just a part of life. If you're reading this, mate, thank you so much; you'll never know how much it meant. We definitely need another game of FIFA so I can settle the score.

While Toby was brainstorming the next part of my treatment, we got to spend a little bit of time at home, and eventually, if I felt up to it, I was allowed to go to school in small increments. I was excited to go and show off my New Year jersey with everyone else. However, there was one small issue in my head: being bald. Sadly, this was not something that I was able to get used to. You'd think that after losing my hair once, I would have become accustomed to it, but this was not the case at all. I was at the age where I cared more about what people think, and I was starting to notice girls a little bit, so being bald in my eyes was the worst-case scenario. The thing is as well – I was so self-conscious about it that I hung on to what was left of my hair. I looked like Homer Simpson; I just had strands of hair on my head. It's quite sad looking back on how desperate I was to keep whatever I had left. This was all that survived from my day when I pulled it out – a few loose strands.

I don't know if I have mentioned it, but I have the best mates in the world. Once again, the boys heard about my dilemma, and they couldn't let me face the battle alone, so on the 16th of June 2015, my mates decided to face the razor again and go completely bald to support me. Before I get into details, I will once again name the boys who did it. There are some familiar names in this crew, as many of them shaved their heads with me the first time as well:

Callum B
Jarvis C
Kai R
Vaughan M
Lachlan W
Kevin H
Reid J
Travis C
Max C
Conor M

Yet again, massive shoutout to these boys – you don't know how much it means to me to have friends who are willing to go above and beyond for me. As my beautiful grandma always told me, 'Tell me who your friends are, and I'll tell you who you are.' The actions portrayed by these boys showed selflessness and kindness on a different level, and this is not just a testament to them but to the people who raised them as well.

You guys should be so proud of your boys; I know my older self is.

So once again, before school, we all packed into a local barbershop, this time in Cronulla for all the boys to get rid of their hair. I'm not sure if they went for a number one last time, but the second time, everyone seemed so much balder. Maybe I was just overthinking it, but they were completely clean-shaven bald. We got a great photo with all of our Year 6 jerseys on and all the boys showing off their haircuts. It meant so much to me, and I appreciated it so much. But still, I refused to get rid of my last few strands. The déjà vu I felt actually was insane; it was almost like we had just been there doing the same thing. This was such a selfless act from all the boys, and I felt blessed that they were there to do it again with me.

This also started a bit of a chain reaction, with a few of my mates that I played footy and cricket with from other schools shaving their heads as well. 2015 would've been a sight to see around the shire, with dozens of kids walking around bald. All jokes aside, though, it's just another example of people coming together to help each other, which truly means a lot. If the world had more of this, it would be a much better place.

As much as the support was awesome from the boys, being twelve years old this time around, I was much more aware of being different, and it was a constant struggle that I had throughout the journey to the second cancer diagnosis. Being the school captain and even just a Year 6 student, I felt as though there were a lot more eyes on me, and I hated being the centre of attention for being 'the sick kid,' especially with how much it made me stand out. I reflected on how much I'd looked up to the older Year 6's throughout school, and when I compared them to myself, I felt weak and not fit for the role. No one made me feel this way or anything; it was just some internal struggles I had throughout the year, and I would rather be completely transparent in my story.

In saying that, it did make going to school the next day a much less daunting task thanks to the boys. They are very special human beings and I will never be able to thank them enough.

After some careful planning (and I am sure a huge amount of pondering), Toby had decided that radiotherapy was the way to go forward, and honestly, I trusted him. It's been a proven strategy for dealing with lymphoma, so it made sense. The new goal was for the radiation to kill the majority of the cancer cells and get me ready for the stem cell transplant. To be eligible for the autologous stem cell transplant, all or most of the cancer cells must not be visible on a PET scan, giving the patient the best chance of survival. Due to the ineffectiveness of the ICE chemotherapy, radiation was now the next step in the treatment plan, hopefully getting me over the line and ready for the transplant.

Very shortly after Toby's orders were in, I went into the hospital to have a planning day, which involved getting everything ready for the radiation treatments. They had to make a custom mask for me to use during the sessions. The mask fit tightly to keep my head perfectly still, which felt pretty intense, but I got why it was necessary. Getting fitted for it was a strange experience. They made a plastic mould of my face that was designed to clip me in place, so I wouldn't be able to move at all during the treatment. It was an odd feeling, having something so rigid and precise on my face, but I understood that it was necessary to ensure everything was lined up perfectly for the radiation. It was just one of those things that felt surreal but made sense in the moment.

It caused me a bit of anxiety being clipped in, as it makes you kind of feel claustrophobic. It was definitely not the most exhilarating thing I've ever done, I can tell you that much. I was also to meet with my radiotherapy oncologist, Dr Robert Smee, who was a lovely man. I remember his grey moustache being very noticeable and him being kind to me, helping my parents and me to calm any nerves. He was very confident in the radiotherapy working, and I was assured by Toby that he was the best in the business. My two oncologists were awesome and both very chill, which was what my family and I needed at the time.

The plan was to start as soon as possible, as I needed to have fifteen sessions spread out over three weeks. Each session would last up to thirty minutes, which doesn't sound like much on paper, but I imagined that it would feel like forever when I was lying there, unable to move. It was just another step forward, another thing to endure, and I kept telling myself it was worth it if it worked.

Despite this, we didn't initially opt for radiotherapy. The long-term side effects can be harsh, including damage to healthy tissue, a long list of potential secondary cancers, and other risks that are hard to overlook. Muscle atrophy in my neck was a major concern, along with the potential for coronary artery disease and damage to my thyroid. Many stomach complications, too, were a risk, as my stomach was set to be radiated too. How can I forget about the short-term side effects as well: burns/blisters around and inside my mouth, stomach pains and nausea. Apparently, it was going to make eating hard (if this wasn't already hard enough).

Radiation wasn't the road we wanted to go down, but at this point, we didn't have any other real options. Occasionally, you just have to take the difficult path and hope it leads somewhere better. I was also keen to have treatment that was going to make me vomit and be sick everywhere (so I thought until my stomach had to get radiated).

Radiotherapy

The first day of radiotherapy was a very nerve-racking day. I remember walking into the Prince of Wales Hospital (next door to my usual Sydney Children's Hospital) and being struck by how surreal the radiotherapy centre was. It honestly felt like something out of a futuristic Star Wars movie. Everything was white, and the whole place had this almost otherworldly, high-tech vibe. My anxiety was at an all-time high, though. I was still consistently suffering panic attacks and shortness of breath from the brentuximab incident. It didn't help either that I had to be pinned down to the bed by my face. I found it really difficult to be anywhere without Mum or Dad around; I hated being alone. Even sometimes waiting in the car or anything, I would freak out and break down in tears as a panic attack would come on, and I would feel like I was unable to breathe.

I knew I was going to struggle with the radiotherapy, as no one else is allowed in the room with you, obviously due to radiation exposure, so I had to try and brave it. This is where I believe I started to become resilient. I began changing the thoughts in my head. I knew it was going to suck, and I knew I'd get anxious, but I realised that if you can change your mindset about a situation, you can change the way you experience it.

I knew I couldn't avoid the tough moments, but by facing them with a different perspective – one that gave me strength instead of letting fear take over – I could get through the challenging times. My anxiety was still going to be there, and I knew I would have a panic attack, but being able to resolve these issues internally without external assistance was something I set myself up to do. At such a young age, I naturally came up with more mature solutions when dealing with stereotypically adult situations like a cancer diagnosis.

I lay down and got strapped in, waiting for the radiation to begin. The room around me was incredibly bright, almost blinding, yet eerily empty, with nothing but the hum of machines filling the silence. I couldn't help but wonder if I would feel any pain or if I would experience anything at all. But to my surprise, the doctors were right. I didn't feel a thing. It was really weird because you hear about how dangerous radiation is; however, it wasn't painful, and you couldn't see it. It's odd how something so dangerous, like radiation, can be completely invisible. There's no sign of it, no way to see or feel its impact, yet you know it's doing its work behind the scenes.

Despite the stillness and the anxious knot in my stomach, I knew I had to face this. So, I focused on taking deep breaths, reminding myself that I could do this. I had no control over the situation, but I had control over how I responded. And at that moment, mindset was everything. 'Deep breaths' was my focus. For the next thirty minutes, it was just deep breaths.

Before I even knew it, I had completed my first dosage of radiation. I immediately became aware of the accompanying fatigue, as it left me feeling exhausted. I was still chatty, though, so that was good; at least I was my normal self. I did notice a red rash developing on my neck, which was a normal side effect of radiation exposure. I was told as well to protect my neck and stomach (where the radiation was going into) from the sun. This wasn't too bad, and I knew that I could do it. One down, fifteen to go.

It became a daily routine, getting ready to go to the hospital and have my radiation therapy. For the first few days, only a rash was occurring, coupled with fatigue, but as the days went on, I started feeling the effects of the radiation. It was about the second week into it when the blisters started appearing around my mouth from the burns. This made eating and drinking an enormous struggle. I also noticed that my mouth was extremely dry; this was normal, as my saliva-producing glands were in the radiation field. The fatigue would get worse, which made going to school a semi-impossible task.

The most I was really getting up to during this period was FIFA. Mum bought me some FIFA points so I could open packs (isn't she the best); as a result, I was opening packs whenever I wasn't at the hospital. I watched a tonne of YouTube as well – just things to pass the time. At the start of my diagnosis, I found it difficult to stay entertained since I was always playing sports or being active. But eventually, the PlayStation became my unexpected companion. It helped me maintain the competitive edge I craved after losing the sports and activities I loved. It wasn't the same as being on the field, but it kept me engaged and gave me a sense of normalcy during a tough time.

Quick story time before I carry on. The Blues were playing their last Origin game against Queensland on Wednesday, the 8th of July. Mic Ennis, the legend he is, pulled some strings and got Trent Hodgkinson to write my name on the kicking tee for New South Wales that game. I was so excited, and Mum and I were at the hospital looking very closely for my name. However, just carrying on with my continued good luck that time, unfortunately, we didn't get to see the tee much at all that game. Some of you may remember that game, but for those who don't, let me fill you in. New South Wales lost 52–6 to Queensland. It was a thrashing! So the tee did not get used much at all. Well, actually, maybe it did with the kickoffs, but nothing close enough to see my name. It was a heartbreaking loss; I must've been the bad luck token. Still to this day it is the biggest Origin loss in the history of the game. How good of a story is that? I reckon that's so funny. So yeah, the moral of the story is don't write my name on the tee; it is bad luck. I do appreciate the thought but, Mic!

Throughout this entire journey, I hope one recurring theme has been the power of helping each other and the invaluable support a community can offer. My family and I were fortunate enough to experience this many times firsthand, with a whole range of people from friends to strangers putting their hand up to help us in any way they could. Up until now, we didn't believe we could find any more support if we tried. However, thanks to one person, everything changed.

A wise man (he'd love that I'm saying this too), named Aaron Raper, decided that he wanted to create a fundraiser for the Sydney Children's Hospital, as they had done such a good job with me. Aaron decided to utilise the infamous shire fundraiser, the Sutherland 2 Surf (S2S) and create the Run 4 Angus to show his support for me, with all the proceeds going towards the children's hospital. He had blue shirts printed with 'Run 4 Angus' in bold black lettering on the front and gave them to everyone who was interested. Aaron had initially planned for about twenty people and aimed to raise a thousand dollars, but he exceeded this goal significantly as over 200 people signed up and wore the shirts. Aaron's son Kai was also one of my good mates, who consistently shaved his head with me both times.

On the 19th of July, the Run 4 Angus race was to take place, and I got up early to meet everyone at the starting line before their run. Let's just say I had zero idea of the sheer number of people who would show up. I can't express in words how loved and supported I felt from this kind gesture. It was crazy to see so many people all come together for me; words can't describe the feeling. Especially seeing a bunch of bald kids (and adults), I couldn't believe it. I have never felt so proud of where I came from; it was inspiring.

This came at the perfect time as I was struggling deeply with the daily radiation treatments. They were taking a serious toll on my body, essentially burning everything in their path. However, Aaron's fundraiser completely took my mind off everything shitty that was going on. Mates from all walks of life like my footy team, cricket team, surf life-saving clubs, you name it, they were there to support me. I had to get front row seats as well for a few of the boys talking a big game about smashing the race, so even though I couldn't compete in it, I still had to be there in the front row to watch it.

I clapped and cheered everyone on as they ran past me. There was a sea of blue shirts, and it was mesmerising to see. Even my schoolteachers came along and ran. It was such a fantastic initiative, and the number of people who told me they don't usually run but made an exception just for the occasion was amazing. I wished I could've been next to everyone running along with them, but this reminded me that things were only temporary, and in no time I would be back. I made sure to keep a close eye on everyone's times so that when I finally did the race, I'd crush their times and have all the bragging rights to rub in their faces!

The S2S is eleven kilometres, which isn't a short distance at all, so for people to run it for me, especially if they didn't run much or didn't enjoy it, was awesome. Everyone gathered at the end of the race to engage in conversation. I got to hear some funny stories from my mates; apparently Jarvis was on Struggle Street, which would've been quality to see. If he ran anything like his FIFA skills, it had to have been a long day for him.

By the end of it all, Aaron ended up raising over $13,000 for the Sydney Children's Hospital, which was an fantastic effort. Massive shoutout again to Aaron and the Raper family for putting on the event. Thanks also to the De La Salle JRLFC and my primary school, Burraneer Bay Public School, communities for getting down there and supporting me. These were just a few of the many incredible people who showed up, and I want to take a moment to thank each and every one of you from the bottom of my heart. Your support, your presence and your kindness meant more to me than words can express. You didn't just show up; everyone came with love and energy and with an unwavering belief that I could make it through. This helped reaffirm my own belief that I could do it, and I'll never be able to fully repay you for what you've done, but I will carry your kindness with me always. Thank you, truly, for being part of this journey.

After an awesome weekend, Monday was straight back to work with the radiation treatments. However, this treatment was different as it was going to be my last on the 20th of July 2015. I was so excited to complete it. The side effects were terrible: my mouth was torn to shreds and I felt very fatigued. In saying this, it was nowhere near as bad as some of the other chemos I have had, but it still wasn't fun. If I had to describe it, it felt like being burned constantly in the same spot every day. That's really the only way I can put it, because burned is exactly what was happening, just a relentless, daily burn that never seemed to stop. Aloe vera didn't even really help either; you just have to kind of cop it. No tan either, which was disappointing, just mostly invisible burns. I mean, if I go through all that, at least give me a tan!

The radiation ward had a bell that you rang whenever you completed your treatment, and I had been eyeing it ever since my first day there. One day, I was sitting with Mum, just minding my own business, when suddenly this loud bell rang. Curiously, I looked over and saw a little boy, grinning from ear to ear as he rang the bell. It warmed my heart at that moment. From that day – about a month ago – I couldn't stop thinking about that bell and the day I was finally going to ring it. Unlike that little boy, my cancer journey was far from over, but the finish line was now in view, and jeez, did it feel attainable.

I left the room after my last treatment with a huge smile on my face. The nurses offered me the radiation mask that had kept me trapped for the past month, and to everyone's surprise (including my own), I decided to keep it. Don't ask where it's gone because I have no idea. I bet Mum or Dad threw it out as they didn't want a reminder, which is a fair point; I would've done the same. Anyways, I marched straight out of the room, thanked the doctors and nurses and B-lined it straight towards that bell. Let me just say the ring I gave that bell, you probably could have heard it in New Zealand. I rang it loud and proud, letting everyone know what I had accomplished. After a fantastic weekend, this day felt like the perfect continuation, one that was just as great, if not almost better. Almost. Mum even let me get KFC on the way home, which was another win. Life was good at the moment, and even though there were so many things going on to bring me down, I wasn't going to let it. A small win is still a win, and sometimes you've got to take what you can get.

A Ray of Hope

Toby had eagerly booked the PET scan for a few days after I'd finished my last radiotherapy treatment. I think he may have been anxious to examine the status of the cancer, and honestly, he wasn't alone; we all were…

All PET scans were incredibly important, but this one was one of the most crucial. There was a tonne relying on this scan; I don't know what the step forward would've been if the radiotherapy didn't work out.

Here I was again, lying in the PET scan machine, an all-too-familiar sight. I couldn't help but reflect on the last time I was here, thinking that my journey was almost over, believing that those hard chemo drugs had done the job, but I was so wrong. As much as the high of finishing my radiotherapy had been at play, the realness of the situation hit me and I was praying there had been a significant decrease in the cancer. I also remember feeling upset then, but it wasn't about my health or the test results. I was fixated on something entirely different: missing out on Year 6 camp.

Ever since I can remember, I had been eagerly looking forward to the Year 6 snow trip. It was the highlight of the school calendar, and every older student I spoke to raved about it, calling it the best camp they'd ever been on. So, when the time came and I realised I wouldn't be able to go, it was devastating. The thought of all my mates returning with all these memories I wouldn't be part of weighed heavily on me. It wasn't just about the snow or the camp; it was about feeling included in something special, something we'd all been anticipating for years.

I had no idea what the future held at that point, and instead of worrying about the medical situation, I was lost in the innocence of wanting to be at camp with my friends. It was strange having the simple, carefree thoughts of a kid coupled with the complexity of what was unfolding in my life. It's exactly what I mentioned earlier: when you're going through something like this as a kid, you're caught between two mindsets. On one hand, you have that innocent child's perspective, where my biggest concerns were things like missing camp or not being able to hang out with my friends. But on the other hand, you're also forced to grow up quickly and maturely handle the situation you've been put in, like difficult conversations, and comprehend the potential horrors of what's happening to your body.

It was a strange and difficult balance to strike, holding onto that childhood innocence while simultaneously carrying the weight of adult realities. I found navigating the two worlds often exhausting, confusing and overwhelming. This, however, ended up helping me a lot as I got older. It made me realise how important it is to prioritise your health and cherish your family time, as well as appreciate experiences like trips and special moments together. If there's one thing about this cancer journey, it is a rollercoaster of emotions. You have to appreciate the highs because the lows are very low, and you can get stuck there. That's why I'm grateful for everything I've experienced so far. As the saying goes, 'Pressure makes diamonds.' As challenging and heartbreaking as it was to face such serious situations at a young age, those experiences gave me the tools to navigate life and strive for success. Everyone has their own struggles, but I truly believe that it's how we face those challenges and grow from them that defines who we are and what we can achieve.

Okay, sorry for the emotional attempt at being inspiring there; I will get back to my story.

Yeah, pretty much that PET scan after the radiotherapy had me in a bit of a weird headspace. I am glad, though, that I didn't let the missed school experiences get me down. Like, if I'm being honest, it did at times, but I kept telling myself it would be bad in the short term and pay off in the long.

The day was finally here to get my results. I use the word 'finally' as if we had been waiting for a long time, but it was actually only a day or two after the scan when we met with Toby to discuss the results and outline the next steps in our plan. Mum and Dad both came again, as they have with all of our big meetings. PET scan results were always hard to get, as the 'Big Dogs' had to score them before any final strategies were made. The 'Big Dogs', as I liked to call them, were kind of Toby's bosses, we will say. They would double-check everything Toby did and make sure that they were the best options for me. Unfortunately, I never got to meet them, but I did appreciate them keeping Toby in line. That was also a joke; Toby was completely fine. I bet it was the opposite way around – he was definitely keeping them in line. Regardless, Toby was more than capable of demonstrating the scan's appearance, allowing us to form judgements based on previous scans. We knew we weren't going to get the full rundown, but all we really wanted to know was how it was looking.

I'll tell you what else: After months of being in and out of the hospital, it was nice coming back to C2North and being an outpatient. We all knew it wouldn't be long before I had the transplant and would spend a tonne of time there, but it was nice just appreciating walking into the hospital with no wheelchairs or hospital beds. A nice change, I must say.

As we sat in the waiting room, I fully remembered the best part about it: the ham sandwiches. They have this little fridge area that is cordoned off so that kids can't get in but being twelve at the time, I could now go in by myself. The rules never changed; it was more just Mum couldn't stop me now. So as we were waiting, I grabbed about three or four of the ham sandwiches. I'll talk crap about hospital food all day, but I will never say a bad thing about those sandwiches. Deadset it was the only thing I'd ever eat in the hospital. Perfect timing too, as my mouth had just recovered from the radiation, so what better way to celebrate?

As I was tucking into my third sandwich, washed down with the off-brand Sprite, Toby appeared to take us to our consultation room. He greeted me with his famous 'Hey, maestro', which always had the same soothing effect on me. Such a simple gesture from Toby, but it actually meant a tremendous amount to me. In a weird way it was soothing, reminding me that I was still a kid, even though at the time, with everything going on, sometimes I lost sight of that. I was trying to get a sense of Toby's mood to see how this PET scan was from his facial expressions or mood. This was a waste of time as Toby is a focused man who barely shows his emotions.

Dad and I used to have a challenge where we could see if we could make him laugh. I can confirm he can laugh, but it's a rare sight. Once I remember him cracking a good laugh when his phone rang, and you wouldn't believe what his ringtone was. This introverted man had the song 'Ground Control to Major Tom' playing when his phone rang. Dad, Toby and I all cracked up when this happened. It was one of the funniest moments, as it was so unexpected. I still can't believe it to be honest, and for those of you asking, we still bring it up with him.

We followed Toby through and sat down in the consultation room. Now what was apparent from the moment we sat down was Toby's smile. This wasn't all too common to see, but it was an amazing sight. Something was good, and after countless meetings that weren't positive, this change-up was just what the doctor ordered, literally. Toby started with his usual chat, which was informative but brief, and then we got into the good stuff. On his computer, he had my previous scan and my new scan next to one another, and what we saw immediately made us join Toby and smile from ear to ear…

There had been a drastic reduction in the cancer cells on the PET scan. Only a few light grey nodes were visible in my neck, and the lymph nodes in my stomach had completely disappeared. This was a thousand times better than my previous scan, where the cancer cells were dark, aggressive nodes that stood out clearly and portrayed the ineffectiveness of the treatment I was having.

Although this was all looking extremely promising, Toby said that we had to wait until Friday to hear the results of the scan and how they were going to grade it. If the grade wasn't at a certain level, I wouldn't have been eligible for the stem cell transplant, so other possible treatment options were going to be explored. Toby always told us everything straight up as he wanted to prepare us for every scenario. In saying that, all of us in that room, including Toby, were confident that the grading was going to be portraying low signs of cancer, and the stem cell transplant was going to be just around the corner.

Our journey home was a good one, filled with laughs and smiles. I was even allowed to go on the aux, which was a rare but exciting occasion. Everything was good. As I've mentioned earlier, celebrate the wins, except this was a massive one, so the celebration was even more meaningful and exciting.

Toby called us back a few days later to fill us in on the results. The meeting concluded that I no longer had active cancer cells in my stomach; however, there was still a small amount of residual disease in my neck. Toby assured us that any remaining abnormal cells would be targeted and 'should' be destroyed with the upcoming intense therapy I was going to have. There are no promises in cancer treatment, so "should" was the best we could expect and we were happy to take it. My second time being sick, the cancer was very stubborn, but this was the best we could achieve before the transplant, and the specialists were confident in moving forward.

Now, I was cleared to go to school for a little bit before the transplant was to start. I was so excited, as I could finally actually participate in my school captain role and hang out with my mates; it had felt like forever. I did have to keep as healthy as possible though, as the transplant was extremely high risk. To have the best chance of everything going smoothly, it was of utmost importance that my body was ready for the torture it was going to be put through.

This chemo regimen was meant to make the ICE protocol look like a piece of cake. Utmost I was also told that the chance of me getting a feeding tube was 100 per cent. I am proud of myself for successfully avoiding it up until this point. My stubbornness saved me, but I was reassured it wouldn't get me much further. I set out a challenge to not get one so we will see how we go (spoilers: I had 0 chance; I was fighting a losing battle).

It was good, though, to have a little bit of relaxation time and go back to a sort of norm. This helped calm my anxiety down, which was very prevalent throughout my second diagnosis. I haven't really mentioned it much after the brentuximab incident, but it was a daily occurrence. I would have panic attacks all the time, and what made it more difficult was the fact that because my friends and I were so young at the time, I felt as though I couldn't talk to them about it. My parents were awesome about it, especially Mum's paramedic friend Paula. She was always happy to calm me down and reassure me that I was not, in fact, dying.

The anxiety was a scary thing, and it made my treatment really hard. I was able to portray to everyone (apart from my family) that I was fine and didn't want to worry anyone about my anxiety and PTSD. I think being around the hospital and always having to stress about the cancer progression, temperatures or anything that these diagnoses came with was just too much to comprehend for anyone, especially for a twelve year old.

Despite everything, as I said earlier, the break before the stem cell transplant was just what I needed to get some normality back into my life: going to school, seeing my friends and just being a normal kid again.

A Touch of Normality

School the first day back was awesome. I did a few half days for the first few weeks, just as I needed some time to readjust. In addition, I was still experiencing the effects of fatigue due to the treatments over the last few months. It was so good to see all my friends again, as my inner circle really became the only faces I saw for a long time. We couldn't risk me getting unwanted germs, as that would've meant another overnight hospital stay. To say the least, we'd had enough of them so it was better to stay on the downlow.

Although it was good to be back at school, the readjustment period was definitely necessary. You'd have to see it to believe it, but even my social battery needed warming up. The fatigue definitely didn't help, but for the first time I found myself turning down hangouts with mates after school as I just needed to rest. However, I want to reassure anyone who knows me that this was only for the first week. Week two was so fun. While I had been away, the boys had discovered some bike jumps just down the road from our school. I'm sure you can guess where this is going.

One afternoon, we all charged down to the jumps to tackle one of the huge new ones that had just been built. As much as I was itching to join in, I knew better than to launch myself off rocks or ramps this time, so I had to pass. I won't lie, I was a bit bummed, but I made the best of it by parking myself under the jumps, daring the boys to soar over me. Looking back, I'm not sure why that seemed like a better option (sorry, Mum!), but hey, at least I made it through unscathed.

Not everyone had the same luck, though. The boys were all over the place with scrapes, bruises and a lot of pride on the line. It turned into this wild competition where each jump had to be bigger and crazier than the last. Someone would hit the biggest jump, and then someone else would be leaping off a rock or something ridiculous. It was exactly as insane as it sounds stupid, sure, but hilarious, and somehow no one got seriously hurt! Kids just being kids, really, and it was cool to experience – completely different from my past few months!

I utilised my time well before the transplant, and I went and watched my old footy and soccer teams. As I got sick before registrations, I never got to register for any winter sports. This was the first year in which I didn't play rugby league or soccer. I was not stoked in any way to be on the sideline, but both of my teams made me feel as though I was a part of it. My old soccer team even made me an assistant coach, which was a great experience. It became clear that, as much as I talk,

I was definitely a better player than coach – I could never take the role too seriously. Coaching was more than likely a one-time thing; maybe when I'm older I'd give it another go, but for now one and done. The things that made sport enjoyable for me were the competitiveness and the feeling of running around with my mates, not telling people what to do from the sideline. It just wasn't my thing. Mum and Dad even took me to a few of the Sharks' home games in my intermission period. Granted, we did stay away from people as I was still immunosuppressed, but it was good to feel normal again and to go and do standard things.

Sometime in the middle of August at our weekly checkup, Toby briefed us on the plan. The 2nd of September 2015 was going to be the day that I started my transplant. He also told us that I had to go into the hospital a week prior, though just for a day, and get a whole range of tests done. These were done to ensure my body could handle the intensity of the treatment and to make sure that my bone marrow would integrate nicely with little to no complications. Blood tests were done to check my blood cell levels and assess how well my liver and kidneys were functioning. I had to get an echocardiogram to check my heart's rhythm, electrical activity and the condition of nearby blood vessels. Lung function tests were measuring how well my lungs were working, while a chest X-ray and CT scan examined the condition of my lungs, liver and other organs.

Back when I was getting my central line put in, I forgot to mention I had a bone marrow biopsy, which involved inserting a needle into my pelvic bone to extract a sample of bone marrow. These results were chased up as they were also needed. I had to provide a urine sample to check my kidney function, and a dental check was done to ensure my teeth and gums were in good shape before treatment. Finally, a bone density scan helped assess the strength of my bones. These tests were all part of preparing me for the challenges ahead. Long day, I know…

Each test had its own specific reasoning for needing to be completed. This was kind of the moment I realised I was getting myself into something drastic, and as close as the finish line seemed, I still had a high mountain to climb. I'm not talking about Mount Kosciuszko; I'm talking about Mount Everest. Was I nervous? Extremely. Was I prepared at all? No. Could I do anything about it? No.

Instead of dreading it, I looked at it like the end. This was going to be the final send-off to a life-changing two years. Although I subconsciously knew these years would change the course of my life, I was determined to go out with a bang and defeat cancer. I refused to let it defeat me or define who I am. The end was near, and I was all for it.

At my primary school, it was a tradition for the Year 6 students to put on a musical as part of their farewell. This was always done at the end of the year. The transplant was perfectly timed for me; if all things went well, I was going to be able to perform in it along with all my friends. This was in around December, so we were hoping that everything went smoothly and I wouldn't miss out. I couldn't contain my excitement when this all planned out; after a year of missing things, I was keen to have my end-of-year celebrations with my cohort – it was going to be awesome. Everything had to go according to plan though first, and there was no confirmation from Toby whether I would 100 per cent be able to do it, but all I needed was that 'it's possible' to get me excited. The trials took place just one day before my transplant was scheduled to begin, specifically on the 1st of September. If I had missed the trials, I wouldn't have been able to go for a main character role, which I would have been devastated about.

This year we were doing the play *Annie*. The play is about a young orphan named Annie, set in 1930s New York, as she embarks on a journey to find her parents. She finds a new family with billionaire Oliver Warbucks, overcoming hardships with hope and determination. The play was a great idea, and everyone in my year was very excited to participate in it. I was not sure what role I wanted, but all I knew is that I wanted to try out and be a main character. The only problem was, for the try-outs, we had to sing in front of the whole year. Let's just say talking is my forte, definitely not singing, and especially not with about a hundred twelve-year-old kids staring at me.

A few of my mates opted out of putting their names down to trial for main character spots as they didn't want to sing, especially not in front of the year. I initially planned to do the same, but then I stopped, paused and reflected on my decision. After everything I had been through this year and in 2013, I wasn't going to do something because I had to sing in front of a large crowd? No way. Even though my friends didn't, I still applied. This goes for anything in life as well. We have all faced challenges and whenever there's something you don't want to do, think about a time you conquered something or overcame a problem you thought you couldn't. Use that as a reminder of your strength and resilience, and take action; you are stronger than you believe.

We have one crack at life, and sometimes it can be horrible, but you can't let it bring you down. My singing was terrible, and it was going to be embarrassing portraying that side of myself in front of my peers, but I wanted the role and wasn't going to let it stop me. We are all far more capable than we realise. Trust me.

I had my eyes set on the prize, the musical, and I knew what I had to do to get there, so it was full steam ahead. My practice regime included one lot of singing in the shower, well, actually, the bath, because I still had the central line in that I couldn't get wet. I'll say this: it's tremendously more awkward singing in the bath, as there is no other background noise to cancel out your terrible singing. By the sound of my singing, too, I didn't know how far I was going to get in these auditions. Hopefully there was a main character role where I didn't have to sing much!

The day of the transplant was approaching quickly. At times, I almost forgot that I was sick, which was a good feeling. Even though I still saw Toby weekly, the days I was at school I was running around and having fun and just being a kid. On the 26th of August, I had all the tests done that I had mentioned earlier. All the results were fine, which was fantastic. Somehow, my fitness was actually better than we anticipated. I was very surprised to see that, and my lungs and heart function were also seemingly unaffected, which was good. Everything else was also fine, which was a bonus. My liver function had recovered from being down for a while, and the same with my kidneys. These were all positive results, and after two years on and off of cancer treatment, this wasn't always a common sight.

Just considering how much the treatment smashes you, we were ecstatic with this. I had the green light, and now nothing was stopping me from having the transplant. It was full steam ahead; I just had to not do anything stupid for the next week, and it was on. I'm hoping by this point in the book you know me well enough. I always have to make everything more difficult, so let's get into the story.

Here we were, one day before my autologous stem cell transplant. A very significant day in many regards, my last day of freedom for a while, and more importantly, the trials for *Annie* the musical. After lunch, the trials were ready to begin, a prospect that excited a few kids greatly. Actually, by a few, I meant the whole year, as we got to get out of class for the last two hours of the day, which was a colossal bonus.

The day began as a typical school day, with nothing unusual happening. I had some teachers and students asking basic questions about the transplant but apart from that, it was just any regular day.

This was until lunch came around. So recently my mates and I had started getting into our tip, but the problem was we could only play on the oval, as the school rule was no running on the asphalt. Just for some context, 'tip' of course referred to when one person is 'in' and had to chase other people down and touch them to make the other person 'it.' Anyway, we, being crazy kids, decided to bend the rules a little bit and play all around the playground, on the grass and on the asphalt. We had been playing for weeks without a single injury, so whenever the teachers told us to stop, we didn't take them seriously. It was just an innocent game in our eyes. They'd always warn us that someone would eventually get hurt on the asphalt, but we never gave it much thought. That was until now.

Crack!

On this yet another fateful day, lunchtime had rolled around, and, as usual, we were playing tip. Before I dive into what happened, let me set the scene with the layout of our school; it'll help with the finer details of the story. The school hall was located near the oval, but to get there, you had to walk down a staircase with about seven or eight steps. After that, there were roughly ten metres of asphalt before you reached the grassy expanse of the oval. It was a very common route to run down the stairs, then get onto the oval to escape from the person who was in for a tip.

On this particular afternoon, I was running away from my mate Jack, who was in. He was much quicker than me and we both knew this, so I had to use my brain and try to evade him. If I'm being honest, if I was using my brain, I would've probably sat down from tip, especially the day before I was meant to go in for treatment (and not to mention being on a strong blood thinner), but we all know that sometimes I don't really think and just go for things.

We were running around the asphalt near the school hall as Jack was closing in on me. I was trying to step and weave, but with no success, as he was getting closer and closer. However, out of the corner of my eye, I spotted the set of stairs leading to the oval. My thought process was that I was more agile than Jack and I could lose him on the stairs and then eventually in the crowd on the oval. Many things were flawed with this idea. First of all, we were both running at full speed; secondly, Jack was a representative soccer player whose strength was both his speed and agility. Honestly, this was all just a recipe for disaster.

In an instant, I took a hard right turn, heading in the direction of the stairs. Jack did the same and was gaining even more ground. As my focus was on my pursuer, I was completely oblivious to my outside surroundings. Before I even had enough time to react, one of the girls in my year came out of nowhere, walking past the stairs. This was not good at all as I was heading straight in her direction; we were about to collide.

I had two options in that split second: collide with the innocent bystander who was peacefully using the stairs as they were meant to be used, or swerve around her and make a desperate attempt to rush down the staircase and carry on with my day. Naturally, I chose option two, because who wouldn't? But let's just say my plan wasn't foolproof. I was moving so fast that 'running' down the stairs turned into something far more dramatic. My feet barely skimmed the steps, and before I knew it, I was airborne, practically leaping from the top step to the very last. It wasn't graceful; it wasn't planned. It was chaos in motion.

CRACK! I hit the ground and rolled a few metres. It took me a few seconds to come to my senses with what had just happened and to gather my bearings. When I did, I straightaway knew that there was a problem. Fortunately, I didn't hit my head or anything vital because that would've been an emergency. Unfortunately, my foot landed awkwardly, twisting to its side in the worst possible way. The momentum of my fall carried my entire body weight down onto it, pinning it beneath me with a sickening crunch. I got up and tried to walk right away, only to realise that my foot was completely numb. Up to this point in my life, I hadn't actually broken any bones, really – maybe a finger or two but nothing drastic – so I had no idea what to expect.

I tried walking a few steps and realised that my foot wasn't giving me much at all. I fell to the ground and gripped my foot as the pain began to intensify, likely after my initial shock had worn off. As much as I want to sit here and act like a hero and say I didn't cry, I won't; I can't lie. The tears came flowing and flowing hard like a river down my face. The terror gripped me. I was more scared than anything else. At that moment, I remembered I was on the blood thinner clexane. The thought hit me like a second blow, making my heart race. What if I was bleeding internally? What if this fall, this stupid, avoidable fall, had caused something far worse? My mind spiralled, the fear far outweighing the pain, even though I like to think my pain tolerance is pretty high. I was always reminded about the severity of even getting a bruise on clexane, so I was kind of freaking out.

By this time, Jack and a few of my mates had grabbed a teacher to come and help me. I took my shoe off to have a look at my foot. Immediately, the size of the swelling became obvious, as my foot looked like a balloon. All the teachers and the school, including myself, knew that we needed to get ice on it ASAP. With the help of a few of the boys and my teacher, they helped me hop up to this office. Mind you, at my primary school, the hall and oval area were at the bottom of a hill, so I'll give myself some credit for making it up to the top, into the office and to the first-aid room.

By the time we were up there, there was already an ice pack waiting for me by one of the teachers, which was good. The quicker we got ice, the less severe the internal bleeding was going to be, as cold is a vasoconstrictor that helps to constrict the blood vessels. Before we even arrived at the office, I had stopped crying and felt more relaxed because my teacher and classmates helped calm me down and reassured me that I would be fine. I was very anxious throughout the whole ordeal, as for months I was told to be careful and not bump myself on anything, let alone fall down a flight of stairs, so you could imagine I was a little distressed.

I got to wait in the vice principal's office with her, which was cool, as she helped to look after me. My primary concern at that point, though, was the *Annie* try-outs. I refused any painkillers and just kept the ice on my swollen foot to ensure that any bruising would subside quickly. The pain was bad though, and it did feel like something was definitely wrong, but my teachers reassured me that they thought I had just rolled it and that it would be fine. They told me to keep ice on it, as they knew that they needed to stop any potential internal bleeding, but apart from that, they said I would be fine. I trusted them and didn't really look into it too much. I don't think they understood the severity of the fall and the fact that I fell down the whole lot of stairs, not just a couple, so I don't blame them for not doing much else. Besides, I wasn't crying and screaming out in pain – not trying to sound like a hero, but I was kind of used to pain.

Plus, there were a lot of painkillers that I wasn't allowed to have, as they would interfere with the boatloads of medications I was on, so we were kind of doing the best we could in the situation. Yeah, I forgot to mention that too. I was on a truckload of medications the whole time during treatment, so we had to be very wary of the things that I took and what I was putting in my body due to the potential for adverse effects. Cancer is terrifying, not just because of the disease, but also due to its many complications. Like the gift that keeps on giving, but if the gifts were terrible. Basically, I felt awful for whoever had to look after me, as it would've been extremely difficult.

By this stage I had been in the office for about an hour. All I could think about was getting to these try-outs. I was not keen to sing at all, but I knew I had to. This play was symbolic of the end of my cancer journey so I couldn't miss my opportunity to participate in a main character role. The teachers weren't too keen on letting me go down to the hall, but let's just say I found out very early that when you are bald, you can be pretty convincing. They wouldn't let me walk down with them; honestly, I don't think I could have walked if I tried, but it was good that I wasn't allowed to. I had to be carried. Yep, carried.

A Year 6 student getting piggybacked down to the hall – how delightful! I am sure you can imagine how embarrassed I was. It was a nice offer and I appreciate my teacher doing it for me. But yeah, look, getting carried into the school hall filled with all your peers looking at you wasn't on my list of things to do today. Let alone all the students I passed on the way down, as I mentioned earlier, the walk wasn't short either. Especially not after making such a scene at lunch. I could've died from embarrassment; I felt my face turning into a tomato. However, not everything was negative; everyone else had to sit on the hard wooden floor while I enjoyed the comfort of my own seat, which felt like a win to me!

Of course, when I came in, everyone came up to my chair to check up on me. I just gave them all a thumbs-up and said, 'It was fine.' I'll reiterate, I knew something more was up, but I was going to the hospital tomorrow to start my transplant, so I just thought we would deal with it then. But, for now, it was time for my audition. I had barely been in the hall two minutes before the teachers called on me to perform my act. I was so distracted by all the questions from my friends that I completely forgot that I had to sing.

The seats were set against the wall, with everyone facing the stage, so I thought I was safe from singing in front of everyone, as I couldn't move because one of my legs was up on another chair beside me. But, to *'make it fair'*, the teachers made everyone turn to face me instead. *Now this is great*, I thought to myself. All the attention had been on me since I fell down the stairs, and now I had to sing in front of everyone with my leg up and my shoe off. It was one of those moments where you could laugh, cry or believe it or not, sing. And you'd better believe I chose singing.

I only had a few seconds to pick a song, and for some reason I went with 'Headlights' by Robin Schulz. I don't understand why I gravitated towards that song, but I did. My mouth moved before my brain could catch up. I thought I'd pick my favourite song, 'Wake Me Up,' by Avicii, but nope, 'Headlights' by Robin Schulz it was.

Now, if you ask me how the singing went, I am going to say pretty good. But look, in all honesty, it was most likely crap. I sang about 30–45 seconds of the song before they said, 'That's all, thank you.' Even to this day, I can't tell if it was because I was good and that was all they needed or if they wanted to shut me up. For the sake of my ego, let's just say they'd heard all they needed from this 'voice of an angel'. And for anyone asking, no, I will not sing for you. I did believe that I hit the high notes well-ish. Yeah, I don't know. All I could do was sit and wait for the results to come out. I was hoping that the foot injury I sustained that day would earn me some sympathy points to help land the role, especially since my singing was more than likely terrible. I guess we will have to wait and see...

Mum and Dad were shocked to get a call that afternoon saying they had to pick me up from the office because I couldn't walk to the car. I couldn't even imagine the stress they must have experienced upon learning that I had injured my foot. They never truly could catch a break, could they? I love you guys. Sorry for all the grey hairs I've caused (Dad)!

The look on Dad's face when he arrived to grab me was priceless. He was in total shock when he walked into the sick bay to come and collect me. After I told him the story, it did stress him out. I did get called 'an idiot', and he did mention that if 'I'd hit my head, it would've killed me'. To be fair, he was not wrong at all, and I definitely was an idiot, but everything was okay (mostly) and we were already being admitted tomorrow so we didn't need any more unnecessary hospital trips.

Luckily I knew an alright physio in Dad and he had a look at my foot. With one little glance he just said, 'Doesn't look too good,' and in Dad's vocabulary that isn't good; it means that it's most likely looking like a fracture or ligament damage. Luckily, since Dad was a physio, we had a bunch of spare boots lying around, so straight away I was placed into a boot and told not to put any weight on it until we found out what was going on. Given the amount of radiation I'd already received, I didn't need any more, since I had reached my lifetime limit; therefore, undergoing unnecessary scans was not advisable.

My foot was extremely swollen and bruised; it kind of spoke for itself in the sense that something was definitely wrong. Mum and Dad were both stressed, as they reiterated the clear instructions from the hospital to 'take care of myself', and here I was now with a busted foot. They were concerned that this might've had an impact on the transplant. I had never considered that possibility before, and once again, they were correct. This would be a serious problem if the transplant got delayed, especially for me and my chances of participating in the school play. In Australia, we have primary school that ends in Year 6, so this was my last year in junior school; next year I would be off to high school. After missing so much, the possibility of being healthy and enjoying the end-of-school festivities felt within reach if all went well with the transplant. Missing out on that was the last thing I needed, especially for my morale, as it was something I was holding onto to help me through the transplant. Now, all we could do was hope that the stupid foot didn't ruin anything, fingers crossed.

The night before my stem cell transplant, Grandma and Pop came down from Moss Vale. They were the best as they'd stepped up a lot to help us when I was sick. Quick shoutout to Pop as well; I look up to him so much. If I can become even half the man he is, I know I'll be a great person. Same as my grandma, as they are just selfless people who put everyone's needs above their own. They are truly exceptional human beings, and I love them so much. I couldn't think of two people

I wanted with me more the night before my transplant than them.

Grandma just made it easier, as she loved to cook, so she made us all dinner that night while Mum, Dad and I got everything set for the hospital. Well, I can't lie, Mum and Dad mostly did everything; I was stuck on the lounge with my stupid foot. They were running around like crazy people grabbing books, blankets, chargers, you name it – they were packing it. We brought UNO and other card games to keep me preoccupied. I was hoping we could steal an Xbox again too. We needed anything that could make sitting in an isolated room just a little more bearable.

I didn't get too much sleep that night. My mind was racing with thoughts, unable to settle down. My parents had kept most of the dreadful information away from me, as my anxiety was terrible by this point of my treatment, especially knowing that I wasn't going to leave the hospital for an extended period of time. Whenever I was anxious, I would place my hand on my heart and try to feel my heartbeat; then my other hand would go on my forehead to feel if I was hot or cold. This was all due to my PTSD. I had seen nurses and doctors perform these checks on me whenever they suspected something was wrong, so I started doing them to myself whenever I felt anxious. Even though I didn't really know what I was exactly feeling for, it helped give me some control.

I think, subconsciously, I missed having some control over my surroundings. While I was sick, Toby and my parents would always make the informed decisions. Obviously this was going to happen as I was young, but it was a weird situation to grasp. I was stuck in the middle, as I wanted to be sheltered so badly and told that everything was going to be okay, but then at the same time my curiosity would get the best of me and I would ask the scary questions.

While I was feeling my head, I came across what I thought was a lump, and just like that, I convinced myself I had a brain tumour. Having been so accustomed to seeing kids with eyes bulging from massive brain tumours or lumps on their heads, I instinctively feared the worst whenever I noticed abnormalities with my body. I pretty much became a hypochondriac because of my anxiety and PTSD, though I had no idea that's what it was at the time. When you're constantly surrounded by the worst-case scenarios a kid can face, it starts to feel like those things are more common than they really are. I had become intimately familiar with not only my cancer but also other cancers, leading my mind to immediately anticipate the worst. So yeah, I became a hypochondriac. I had lost complete trust in my body.

This is what was going through my head the night before I was set for the transplant. As much as I tried to not wake up Mum and Dad, I couldn't help but think of myself having a brain tumour, and it all became too much. Although I was such a positive kid, I always still had my fair share of dark days, where I let my anxiety get the best of me, and this was one of those times. I tried to not let anyone know about these days, as I acknowledged how much stress everyone was under already, and they didn't need this on top of it. If I could keep it to myself, I would. These times were all a normal part of the process, but I hated being like that. I wanted to be known as being positive and always happy.

I ran out of my room and woke up Mum and Dad in tears. Not once did I think about my destroyed foot; I just felt so scared. I was extremely emotional; the past year had been challenging, and I often felt as though I would never recover. Mum and Dad managed to calm me down, as they always do, not by convincing me I didn't have a tumour (my mind was already set on that), but by reassuring me that we'd be at the hospital tomorrow to get it checked out. That was the reassurance I needed to get through the night. I slept in the bed with them that night. Again, I'd love to be a hero and say that this wasn't common, but it was very common when I was at home to sleep in their bed with them. Even at twelve years old, I know it's embarrassing to admit, but they just made me feel safe, like nothing would ever happen to me if they were there.

Their cuddles were filled with love, and it helped ease my mind enough to get me to sleep. Tomorrow was a big day: the transplant was finally happening, and I needed my rest. That's why being curled up in my parents' bed helped me feel comfort and a bit of peace before everything began. A month from hell was upon us.

Isolation Month Begins

Just briefly, before I get into my autologous stem cell transplant, I just want to pre-emptively warn everyone that once again these were some of the darkest days of my whole sickness journey. I was struggling massively with anxiety, PTSD, loneliness and a handful of other things. I was so young, but I knew so much that I was fearful of everything. But with my youth came the misunderstanding of statistics and percentages and even simple things like risk-to-reward scenarios. This stem cell transplant was an incredibly high-risk procedure, with countless ways for things to go wrong, especially since the chemotherapy would wipe out everything, obliterating my immune system and leaving me utterly defenceless against even the smallest threat.

I just wanted to quickly apologise for the drop in mood, as this part isn't going to be fun, and I like to keep everything positive. But, as I said from the start, I want to be completely transparent with everyone and honest and open about my journey, just to show that not everything is always going to be sunshine and rainbows, and you will have dark days. But those dark days strengthen you and make you appreciate the better days.

P.S. Some days will be brief with little explanation, simply because there were days I slept through entirely. I was so unwell most of the time that sleep was all I could manage…

Day 1

After a restless night, to say the least, the day had come. I was due in the hospital at around ten a.m., so we didn't have to rush there first thing in the morning, which was good. This time was vital for me, as I got to spend it with my grandparents and siblings. They were excellent at distracting me and making sure that I was okay. Henry even brought Eddie (my cat at the time) to sit with me while Mum and Dad were getting ready. I wasn't much help, as my foot today looked terrible. The swelling was still huge, but this time it was accompanied by terrible bruising. My foot was definitely not sweet, but we were going to the right place to get it checked out.

Mum had called the hospital and briefed them about our unfortunate situation. No one could believe it; the day before a stem cell transplant and I'd physically injured myself. 'This hasn't happened before,' Mum was told. We were relieved, though, when the nurse assured us that it wouldn't affect the transplant.

Grandma, being Italian, loves to cook. I was extremely nervous and not eager to have any food. Not under Grandma's watchful eye, though. She makes the best bacon and fried eggs and she always insists on making sure I eat a proper meal, especially when she sees me looking tentative. I couldn't help but smile at her determination to feed me, even if my appetite wasn't cooperating. The eggs were perfect, and the bacon was crispy. Somehow, under her watchful eye, I found myself savouring every bite. Grandma has a way of making food taste like love. She could tell I was nervous, but she didn't say a word about it. Instead, she set my breakfast down in front of me with a warm smile and followed it up with a big, comforting hug. Although at this point everything was up in the air, it made me feel like everything was going to be okay.

I hugged my family and cat Eddie for the last time, and then we set off for the hospital. I knew the boys were going to be in good hands with Grandma and Pop looking after them, and there was definitely some jealousy on my end.

We ended up leaving the house earlier than anticipated so that we could get an X-ray for my stupid foot. Dad had to carry me into the car. I am acting like this was a giant task, but I was literally about thirty-seven kilograms at this point. There was not much of me at all, just skin and bone.

The car ride felt strange, like we were heading into the unknown. None of us really knew what to expect, and the quiet tension in the air made it feel like we were embarking on some kind of mission. The roads seemed emptier than usual, or maybe I was just too focused on the knot of nerves in my stomach to notice much of anything.

When we finally pulled up to the hospital, Dad dropped us off at the entrance. A wheelchair was waiting for me, which felt weirdly official, like I was suddenly the main character in some dramatic story. It was kind of cool, though, having a chair ready just for me. It made the whole thing feel both serious and surreal at the same time. I have used a wheelchair a few times, but those instances occurred when I was physically unable to walk and extremely unwell. This time, it was all because of my stupid actions. When I saw the wheelchair waiting for me, I couldn't help but think of my older brother Henry. He used to love it when I had to use a wheelchair; he'd take it for joyrides around the hospital, zipping through hallways and trying to do wheelies. The memory made me chuckle quietly to myself as I was wheeled straight to the radiology department.

The radiographer mentioned, as he was setting up the X-ray machine, that my foot looked good. He exclaimed how he 'couldn't be certain, but it definitely looked fractured.' I appreciated his honesty, and it helped to settle my mind. All this fussing over my foot helped me to forget about the brain tumour that I was convinced I had, which was good. After my X-ray, they sent us up to my room, which would serve as my home for the foreseeable future.

I was placed into bed 18, which would be my comfortable little home for now. Lots of cupboard space and a fridge were the main few features that were worth mentioning; the rest was just a bland, plain old hospital room. Luckily, I had a little window to allow some sunshine to pass through, otherwise the room would've been dark and cold. I glared outside at the free world, people walking around and kids playing. I found it hard to comprehend that this is what it had come to, but I knew that this final push was going to get the job done.

Mum made sure to place all my stuff into the cupboard. She ended up packing my Cronulla Shark's pillow, which was a necessity, helping me through the difficult times. The chemo was going to start tomorrow, so today was just really all about getting settled in my new home.

Not long after we unpacked everything, a nurse from radiology came up to deliver the news. So it turns out I didn't break one bone. I broke three. Yep, that is correct, three bones. We were in shock. No wonder my foot was so swollen. I thought maybe one little fracture but no. The nurse informed us that I was to be in a boot for six weeks. I was always non-weight-bearing for two, but as I said earlier, there was zero chance I was going to be able to walk around for a while, so I guess it was the best time for this to happen. I thought to myself, *I gave it a good crack. And if I was going to break something, I might as well go all in with three fractures for good measure.*

I had to ensure my leg was elevated, so I went straight to bed to rest it. My anxiety was at an all-time high, though. I was very fearful of what was to come. The lump on my head also caused me a great deal of worry. Even when the nurse reassured me it was quite literally just my skull, I was still anxious and felt like I was going to have a panic attack all the time. I was stuck in a weird mindset, as I knew so much about what was going on, but at the same time, compared to my parents, I knew nothing. This caused me a greater deal of anxiety, but it was hard. Do you tell me more, or leave it at what I know? It would've been difficult for Mum and Dad. No matter what you're going through, I wholeheartedly believe it's so much harder on the people you love. They are also experiencing the battle, but they are looking in from the outside, trying to assist in any way they can.

Apart from the X-rays and getting all settled in my room, there was not much else exciting that happened on day one. Tomorrow was the big day in which I started my chemotherapy. I needed to get a good rest and try to relax as well as I could because the next few days were big days and I needed as much rest as possible. I had to get used to hospital food again, which was a bonus! Luckily for me, across the road was a Chinese restaurant, and I love Chinese. Whenever I felt hungry, I was fortunate to have parents who would try their best to get me what I wanted, as any food was the goal. I loved the satay chicken, so best believe to get me through the transplant, there would be a tonne of satay chicken.

Mum stayed by my side that night in the pullout lounge. I wish I'd appreciated it more what they put themselves through, as those beds were terrible. But without fail every single night, Mum or Dad would sleep next to me, making me feel safe and ensuring that nothing would happen to me. It made me feel invincible. I remember even saying a prayer that night, 'Look after my family and friends and say hi to Baz up there, and I hope I am making him proud.' You might expect that I would have mentioned the importance of looking after myself, but my parents and family provided me with a sense of safety. Despite the traumatic memories that continued to haunt me and the panic attacks I experienced, having Mum and Dad by my side made me feel capable of conquering anything. Plus, saying a prayer sometimes also comforted me, so I stuck to what I knew. These were my last thoughts before I drifted off to sleep. Once again, it was a restless night, with not much sleep involved, but as I said, focusing on the positives was the way forward, and this was the beginning of the end…

The Long Haul

Day 2

The wake-up for my first full day in the hospital was terrible, as I was incredibly anxious. I didn't feel ready at all for what the day was bringing. Remember at the start of my story I briefly mentioned how I had chemotherapy that was derived from mustard gas? Well, this was the day. Carmustine was its name, and yes, it was an ingredient used in the deadly gas during World War Two. Fun fact: This was actually how its anti-cancer properties were discovered as an agent during the war. This was cool and all, but I was also at the age where I could use Google. It didn't help one bit with my anxiety, as with every chemo drug I could, I would look up the drug and read up on the side effects. I'm sure you can imagine that most of the side effects were not the slightest bit good, which entirely freaked me out.

I was incredibly anxious, and the minutes were stretching longer than they should. Even before the chemo had started, I was petrified. Not only that, but I kept calling the nurse every five minutes, convinced something wasn't right. As usual, my blood pressure was low, and I sensed a creeping discomfort in my body, but I couldn't determine if it was genuine or just a figment of my mind.

I knew too much and not enough at the same time. I had read about every possible side effect, from the mild to the life-threatening, and my brain had latched onto the worst ones. The knowledge was supposed to make me feel prepared, but all it did was fuel my anxiety. My body was a battleground between logic and fear, and fear was winning.

The nurses were very patient, despite the circumstances. They reassured me, checked my vitals, and tried to keep me calm. But the waiting was unbearable. I wanted them to speed up the process, to confirm that I wasn't dying. Because of the brentuximab reaction, I would go into full panic mode whenever I encountered any new drug or substance entering my body, as if I were experiencing an anaphylactic reaction to that drug. So the time before the chemo was even administered, I just spent it freaking out and being fearful of what was to come. It was a very dramatic time, and it would've been draining for everyone involved.

We had to try and get my blood pressure back up before I could even start the chemo so that it would be 'safe' enough to have. This involved pumping my IV full of fluids and getting me to eat some food. I was so anxious that I didn't want

Mum leaving my side. Even leaving me for a couple of minutes to get some food from the fridge would just cause me to panic.

The fear I had about this whole process was overwhelming, but I knew I had to get it done. I just had to have the chemo for five days straight, and then that was it. For the rest of my life, I was trying to look at it through this scope and break it down instead of seeing the gigantic mountain that I had to climb.

You'd think that after seeing the chemo wheeled in so many times with nurses covered head to toe in protective gear, I'd be used to it. But that was never the case. If anything, it felt like they were even more cautious than usual. Then again, when one of the ingredients was once used in deadly gas during wartime, you wouldn't want it getting anywhere near you, would you?

The nurses were actually really awesome and stayed with Mum and me for the first bit of the transfusion. They were most likely just making sure the start of the transfusion was going smoothly and I had no adverse effects to the chemo, but it made me feel safe. Having Mum there would especially make me feel safe and that I could get through it. This set the tone for the rest of my stay. Once the chemo started, it hit me that I didn't even realise that that was the last time I would see the nurses not covered in the protective gear. From now on, the nurses had to be fully covered in masks, gloves, and everything whenever they saw me. As my immune system was about to drop to zero, even the smallest germ could be life-threatening.

I felt very isolated, in the sense that the only people I'd see without full PPE the whole time would be my parents. Everyone else had to treat me like I was toxic because I quite literally was.

The chemotherapy transfusion didn't take that long, which was a positive, but whether it took five hours or five minutes didn't change much out of my day. They were also draining sessions for me as well, as I would make sure I watched the transfusion myself.

I learned about the danger of air bubbles getting into my bloodstream back in 2013 when I was first in the hospital. I was with Dad, who had been a nurse for a very brief period when he was young, and he knew a thing or two about health and hospitals. One night, only a few days after my biopsy surgery, I was in bed and Dad noticed my IV line was filled with air. A little bit of air bubbles wasn't an issue, but his wasn't the case. There were dangerous amounts of air in my line, so Dad stopped the drip and fortunately called the nurse to come and fix it. This wasn't good and although Dad never went into too much detail about it, it always stuck with me. So from then on, whenever I had a transfusion going on, I would check and make sure there were no air bubbles in my drip. This would mean that unless I was asleep, I was inspecting every inch of the line to make sure I would get no air bubbles. I would refuse to do anything else, as I would be anxious until I knew I had made sure that there was no air going into the drip. This took up the majority of my chemo session, so when the final beeping came to indicate the chemo had finished, I now had to find something else to do.

My options were pretty limited. It was either A: lay in bed or B: sit in the chair next to my bed. Both were very stagnant activities and neither would be fun, but what else could I do? Plus, it usually took a few hours before the side effects of the chemo kicked in, so for now it was just chill time and watch TV.

I always found I would be exhausted after the chemo sessions, and day two was no exception. I think that stressing for multiple hours would just drain my body and make me exhausted.

The rest of the second day was resting and watching TV. One of the most eventful days that had come, not in a good way though, was just my anxiety being so high during this period. Little did I know it was only going to go downhill from here. There was a long journey ahead of me.

Day 3

The fatigue had already hit me, and it was only the second full day. It's crazy to see how much chemotherapy can affect you, especially in a short time span. I had almost forgotten about how I felt after it, as I hadn't had chemo since the ICE protocol all those months back. The sleep was good, but not in like I felt well rested; it was more like I was just knocked out.

Today was day two of the chemo, and much like yesterday, I was very nervous. However, Mum told me that there was a surprise for me this afternoon on the Starlight TV station. I was confused, but very excited, as I had no idea why they would be mentioning me. I also forgot to mention that the Starlight quiz was one of the few things I looked forward to during my long stay. Every night at 6 p.m. the quiz would be on, and best believe I would make sure that I was one of the first callers to get involved.

I had that to look forward to, so I just had to get through today. At that moment, I realised I worked best when I had a goal – something to look forward to. Even small wins, like being featured on Starlight TV, gave me purpose. But to reach that goal, I had to go through chemo. It was a brief period of suffering that ultimately led to a rewarding moment. If I could endure the hardship, I'd earn the reward in the end. I liked to think of it like that, and I decided that each day I would try my best to have a little something to look forward to, which would keep me pushing through the harder times. I liked this philosophy and decided to live this way through the next rough period. (What I didn't know was that this idea would be used throughout my entire life, and I still use it to this day).

Today's chemo was going to be etoposide. This was another strong chemotherapy drug that would be added to the cocktail aimed at reducing my immunity to zero. I was not keen at all to have chemo again, but what can I say? What can you do? The nausea hadn't quite hit yet, although my appetite was starting to fade, and it faded quickly. I didn't know whether it was the hospital breakfast or the chemotherapy. Let's just say it was a blend of both.

I was starting to get into the routine of everything now; each morning the nurses would take my blood pressure and temperature at around seven. Then, breakfast would arrive around eight. I'd usually spend a few minutes trying to figure out what was in front of me. I'm just kidding; I know the hospital staff worked hard to feed us. Between the early hours of nine to ten a.m., a crew of oncologists and doctors would come around and visit me to pretty much brief us and tell us the plan moving forward for the day. Toby would even make some celebrity appearances, which would cheer me up. It was always good reminding him how terrible the Manly Sea Eagles were – a great start to the day.

By around lunchtime was when the chemotherapy would arrive, and as I said earlier, it was another new treatment for this day. I actually didn't look up too much about etoposide, but I knew enough about the other chemos, and I had heard enough about what these transplant chemos were trying to do to know that this wasn't going to be fun.

Same old process: The nurse walked in dressed like I was the most toxic thing on this planet, put the chemo bag up, double-checked that I was the correct patient and it was go-time. This day I actually felt the fatigue and I did sleep a lot. But it was only going to get worse. There were positives and negatives to this, though. The positive was that when I was sleeping, I was not anxious and freaking out, which was a huge relief for myself and everyone around me. The negative, though, was the more I slept, the less and less food I was eating. The less I ate, the quicker the feeding tube was going to come. My goal was to completely avoid it, but with more sleep and less eating, the chance of my getting one was becoming more and more likely.

The oncologists and doctors checked my weight every day, so if they noticed a steady drop in kilograms, I wouldn't have much choice but to get the feeding tube. This was a scary reality that I knew I could control, but I felt so tired, even a little bit nauseous actually, after I woke from the etoposide chemotherapy. I knew, too, that when the nausea came, it was not going to leave for a long time. This wasn't good.

However, in positive news, I woke up just in time for my surprise that was waiting for me on the Starlight TV. I was featured in Starlight TV's top 5, which was awesome. The show highlighted the kids who had been actively participating in the quizzes and were performing well, either by winning or scoring a lot of points. They called me on live TV and I got to speak to Captain Starlight himself! It was such a brilliant experience; I had a prize delivered to my room, and they showed pictures of me on the television. I thoroughly enjoyed it, and it put a huge smile on my face for the rest of the day. Things like this were the perfect distraction and just what I needed.

I barely touched dinner, and as much as I was reminded about the feeding tube, I was starting to feel sicker and sicker, and less like eating.

I enjoyed the nighttime a lot more than the daytime. This was due to one thing and one thing only: The quality of the shows on TV was so much better at night. Even Starlight TV had quality kids' movies on at night, which were good. At night either Mum or Dad, depending on who was there, would come up and lay next to me on my bed, and we would watch TV together. As much as the hospital was terrible, I really appreciated this time with Mum and Dad. Mum was still there with me at this point, but I just remember us sitting up and watching some TV. Although I was nauseous, this was a good night. I went to bed happy, with little to no anxiety, which was a nice change. I was enjoying myself as best as I could; however, with the hospital, you never knew what was around the corner.

New Routine

Day 4

Yeah, the nausea had definitely hit me; there was a bit of vomiting through the night, and I was starting to feel real crap. The worst part was that this was just the beginning of the vomiting. On this particular morning, however, I received a photo from my soccer team, the 12Bs, who had sent me an update on how they were all doing. It was nice to see them thinking of me, and it made me smile. It felt good to be remembered, as it would've been so easy to forget about me because I was not present at all.

Who would've guessed it? By this point, another day of chemotherapy was in front of me, and I just had to get it done. Ara-C, also known as cytarabine, was the name of the chemotherapy medication this time. Now, this was one of the heavy chemos that was directly meant to suppress and kill my immune system. Although all the chemos were heavy, this had a direct correlation with wiping out my white blood cells and stem cells. Remember when I said I 'felt sick' before? That experience was insignificant compared to what I would endure after receiving cytarabine. Unfortunately, this was the beginning of a steep decline. The nurse arrived with the chemo, and I watched as they carefully hooked it up to my line.

Mum was going home today to get some rest, as I'm sure you can imagine that sleeping on a small hospital pullout chair for multiple days on end would be exhausting. It would be particularly taxing to care for a sick child who was prone to frequent panic attacks. Dad had come in instead and was to stay with me for a few days.

The process, after enough times, had now just become a routine. Although it was a daily occurrence, it still didn't make it any easier. I felt a little nervous; I knew that this one was strong. I knew that a difficult moment was about to hit me hard so I took a deep breath and tried to settle down, reminding myself that I just had to get through it. One more round. One more step forward. 'There are only a few more days left of chemo forever,' I said to myself. It was weird to think that, and I know there are no guarantees, but this eased my young mind at the time.

As the chemo started dripping into my body, I felt the familiar cold sensation spreading through my veins. I hated that feeling. Although it wasn't painful, the feeling unnerved me, serving as a constant reminder that this poison intended to obliterate parts of me in order to sustain my life. This time, the nurse stayed for a little while to monitor me before leaving me to rest. I appreciated it when they waited for me, just making sure everything was good. It made me feel safe.

At this point, I was not hungry at all, which was not a good sign. Dad pushed hard to try and get me to eat something, but I couldn't. After the chemo, I was just smashed, and all I wanted was to sleep. I felt my eyes getting really heavy. Not long after, the exhaustion crept in and overcame me. The nausea that I had felt for the past few days was lingering from the night before, but at this point, I was too tired to care. This was a good sign, as even though I was nauseous and felt unwell, if I were really sick, my body wouldn't care if it was tired or anything; I would just vomit everywhere. My body did, however, feel fragile. The only thing I could do was close my eyes. Before I knew it, I had drifted off into a deep sleep.

Apart from Dad coming in, it was a very uneventful day four. The days were beginning to all blur together. I had only been here a few days, but the repetitiveness of the routine was already wearing me down. Each day felt the same: blood tests, medications, chemo, sleep, repeat. It was challenging to stay motivated when every moment blended into the next.

I had to keep going forward though, and every day that passed was a day closer to freedom, and damn would it be sweet.

Day 5

Today was actually Father's Day, and where else would Dad have liked to spend it than in the hospital with me! All jokes aside, I hope Dad had a good day and I showed him how much I appreciated him.

More chemo was on the forecast for today. After this round, I had two more days to complete the intense regimen. On the schedule for today was melphalan, another heavy-hitting chemo. As of now, you will notice the pattern that all the chemos in the transplant were heavy-hitting. The effects, even though they weren't great now, over the next coming weeks I was going to really feel it, so this was still almost like the journey hadn't really started. They were tracking my blood, attempting to drop my white blood cell count to zero.

On day seven, my stem cells would be injected back into me. We were starting to get briefed on what to expect. The oncologists and doctors referred to that day as the official 'Day One', the moment my stem cell graft would take place. It was a little disheartening to hear that technically these days didn't count, as I hadn't received my stem cells; this was just really preparing my body for the process. Weird to think that to prep me, they had to kill pretty much everything in my body. I thought of it like a reset.

The Sharks were versing Manly that night, so I'm sure you can imagine how much I wanted the Sharks to win, especially as Toby was coming in to see me tomorrow. If the Sharks won, I doubt that Toby would have heard the end of it. This also gave me something to look forward to in the afternoon, after the chemo was wrapped up.

Same time, same place, the nurse in all her gear came in to give me my chemo. Another bag of poison dripped into my veins. By this point, the routine was second nature: nurses in protective gear, the cold sensation in my arm and the beeping machines. Seven straight days of this, and yet, each day felt harder and harder than the next.

My eating and drinking had been slowing down drastically over the past couple of days. I was still trying to eat and drink, but it was becoming more and more of a struggle. Sleeping all the time was gradually becoming the norm for me as I felt more and more exhausted every day. The constant beeping of my pumps would fill the room. This was a never-ending reminder that something was always being pushed into my body. Whether it was chemo, fluids or medication, the alarms would go off, sometimes in the middle of the night, jolting me awake, and other times blending into the background like white noise.

Just before the chemo was about to finish, I started to spiral. At that moment, I became painfully aware of my situation and that I couldn't escape it. I looked up at the pumps attached to me, now feeling like they were a part of me, a constant reminder of my reality. It was frustrating. I wanted to move freely, but every step, every shift, was a process. Even in my sleep, I had to be careful not to roll onto the lines or set off an alarm. It made me feel even more like a prisoner.

It was still early days, yet every moment felt like a battle. Dad could see how much it was getting to me, and he sympathised. Having him there helped, especially because, like me, he had always been active and understood how hard it was to be stuck in one place. He reassured me, saying, 'We're in this together.' That helped calm me down, at least for a little while.

Sunday afternoon footy was the perfect distraction for me and a good opportunity for Dad and me to celebrate Father's Day as best as possible. The mighty Cronulla Sharks vs. the Manly Sea Eagles, the battle of the beaches – I was excited.

The game was a very close, back-and-forth. Both sides fought valiantly, I'll say, but there could only be one winner. I had waited all day for this, and unfortunately the winner wasn't the Sharks. Manly won 14–12. I was not keen to see Toby; although he didn't speak as much as I did, he definitely wouldn't let me live this down.

After the game, I felt my eyes grow heavy. I tried to fight the fatigue, but there was no use; my body had already decided for me. That was all she wrote for my fourth day of chemo.

Day 6

Another day, another dollar. Today was my second last day of chemo, and I could see the finish line (of chemotherapy; I still had a lot of days in isolation). I was very excited, but I didn't get to show too much of it. I was now feeling the fatigue throughout my whole day. I would wake up tired and want to go back to sleep. This made eating and drinking impossible.

When the oncologists and doctors came and visited me in the morning, they raised concerns about my weight, as I had lost a substantial amount. They said if I didn't do anything today, I would be getting a feeding tube. During this week, they had been giving me electrolytes and food alternatives through my central line. This wasn't substantial at all, and they needed the space on my line for others, like medications and fluids. I had no choice, really, but I didn't want to give up. I told them that I would eat lots of food today and I wouldn't need the feeding tube.

Furthermore, I was struggling badly, but I didn't want to give up; there was no way I was getting one of those tubes. The thought of it even gave me anxiety, especially when they explained in detail how the tubes work. This was meant to calm my nerves, but explaining how it worked sounded horrible. I couldn't see how this would've made me want to correspond. I had a day to prove myself; let's see how I'd go.

I tried to eat, but the moment the food was in front of me, I felt my stomach turn. The sight, the smell – everything about it made me feel worse. I wasn't hungry at all, not even a little. I knew I needed to eat, but the thought of swallowing anything felt impossible. Every bite sat heavily in my mouth, my body rejecting it before I even had the chance to chew. I tasted defeat, and I knew that the inevitable was coming; there was nothing that I could do. The feeding tube was on its way.

The transplant team told us that they also wanted the hospital teacher to come and give me a visit. This probably wasn't the worst idea, but at that time, while I was feeling extremely sick and fatigued, the last thing I wanted to do was sit and try to learn things. However, as I mentioned before, as terrible as I felt, it was only going to get worse. Her name was Cassie, and she was very friendly. I had met her before. This was probably good for me, as all I had been doing was watching *The Simpsons*, a great show, but not the most educational.

Cassie arrived just after midday, a short time after they had put my chemo up. Today was more mustard gas (carmustine), which sounded fun. Multiple days of chemo treatment were definitely beating me, and this day was no better. But, I will say it was nice working with the hospital teacher to help take my mind off things and bring a sort of normality. Far from normal, I know, but I remember something about this day being more positive whilst I was learning, which was odd, but hey, a win's a win. Dad sent Mum a photo of me with Cassie, and let's just say Mum was very excited. This made it that little bit more worth it, hearing Mum was stoked that I was learning. We did some math and English. Cassie was also surprised to find out that I read books. I used to love books; reading would just allow me to escape whatever situation I was in and hone in on the story.

Cassie stayed for just shy of an hour before I could no longer handle the mental strain and started to fall asleep. One more day of chemo tomorrow, and then I was getting the transplant the following day. I was taking small steps towards a bigger goal.

Goodbye, Chemo
Hello, Stem Cells

Day 7

LAST DAY OF CHEMO! I wasn't that excited; it was just a big milestone. At the time, I thought that this was going to be my last ever chemotherapy treatment. As much as I wished that I was pleased and thrilled, I was feeling really crook and anxious. I hadn't eaten all week, and as much as I tried to get stuff down yesterday, I was struggling. The weakness I was feeling made it hard for me to get out of bed, which in turn caused me to feel more anxious and panic. My body just felt horrible. Every day had been the same: chemo after chemo, IV bags switching out like clockwork, and the nurses covered head to toe in protective gear while pumping poison into my body. I knew it was meant to help me, but it didn't feel that way. It felt like I was being stripped down to nothing, every ounce of strength and normality taken from me.

During these times, I didn't like looking at myself as I felt so terrible. I didn't want to see who was looking back at me in the mirror; I could barely recognise him. It would make me sad to see what I had become, and I couldn't understand. I knew I was sick and everything, but it was still so weird looking like a cancer patient. I used to just reflect on how only a year ago I was just a normal kid again, running around playing with my mates, enjoying my life. Now I was locked in the hospital, with no escape for the time being. Crazy how life works sometimes, isn't it? You have to be grateful and appreciate the good days.

Well, I must've looked as horrible as I felt, as without hesitation, when the oncology team came to do their round, I was told I had to get a feeding tube today; there was no more discussion to be had. They knew I tried hard yesterday to get food down, but enough was enough. The last thing they needed was another concern about my lack of nutrients. There was already more than enough to worry about. I understood and respected their decision, but I was so nervous and anxious it was not even funny. The day I had dreaded for so long had finally arrived, and I could no longer avoid it: Feeding Tube.

I had tried to strike a deal with them to wait until the chemo was finished before inserting the feeding tube. It was my way of clinging to some control, stalling it for as long as I could. You wouldn't believe it, but that day was the first and only time in my life that I didn't want the chemo to end.

That's how much I hated the thought of the feeding tube. I was willing to sit through the treatment, through every drop of poison, if it meant avoiding that stupid thing. However, as much as I pleaded, they were not keen. They were firm but fair, pointing out that I could have had it installed days ago, but they were giving me a pass because it was causing me so much anxiety. It was getting installed this morning and there was nothing I could do about it. My heart sank, with a thousand thoughts running through my mind.

The story of my feeding tube insertion goes as follows. There are many parts of my cancer journey that are blurry; however, I remember this like it was yesterday. It has scarred me and I will forever reflect on this moment with goosebumps and shivers…

The nurse walked into the room carrying the tube. I wanted to get up and run, but there was nowhere to go. It was time and I couldn't do anything about it. I sat on the hospital bed, my whole body tense.

A nurse came up and explained the procedure to me. She was a lovely lady and reassured me that everything was going to be okay. As she stood beside me and explained everything, I couldn't help but notice her emphasis on keeping on swallowing. It made me scared, as I didn't want the stupid thing in my lungs. I always feared the worst, and I thought it would happen to me. She was very honest with me, and when I asked the scary questions, she would answer them. Like, there's a chance it could give me life-threatening pneumonia if it happened to get in my lung. I was told that she'd only accidentally had the feeding tube go in one or two people's lungs before… That was all I needed to hear before I started properly freaking out.

It was time. I saw her approaching, holding the thin plastic tube that was about to be threaded up my nose and down my throat. My chest tightened with fear. I knew I had no choice, but that didn't make it any easier.

'Head back,' the nurse instructed gently.

I reluctantly obeyed her, tilting my head back as far as I could. I swear you could've heard my heartbeat in that room as it was thumping so loud. The moment the tube touched my nostril, I winced. It felt so unnatural and just purely wrong. Slowly, she began to push the tube down my throat and instantly, my eyes started watering. I was feeling like I was about to vomit. My nose was on fire, and I had an uncontrollable urge to sneeze, but all I could do was sit there and try to keep swallowing. Everything in my body wanted to get out of there, but I couldn't

'Swallow,' she said. 'Keep swallowing.'

I tried. I really did. But every time I swallowed, I felt the tube dragging against the back of my throat, inching its way further down. I just couldn't stop thinking about where it was ending up. My mind was racing with the same questions: Was it in my throat? Or my lung? What if it went the wrong way? What if I choked? My mind raced with panic. I was supposed to be breathing through my mouth, but I was struggling to breathe, as I was so concerned with making sure I continued to swallow.

Tears began to stream down my face. It wasn't just the physical discomfort; it was the overwhelming feeling of the tube slowly going down my throat. I just wanted it to be over. This felt like eternity, like it was never going to end.

Finally, after what felt like forever, the nurse secured the tape to my cheek, fixing the tube in place. It was finally over. However, my first thoughts were not the feeling of relief the nurse said I would feel. I could still feel it at the back of my throat; it just kept making me gag. She assured me that it would go away soon, but I didn't believe her. I couldn't stop feeling it sitting there.

I wiped my eyes, but the tears kept coming. I actually couldn't stop crying; the experience was one of the worst of my young life. My chest felt so tight, and my body couldn't stop shaking from the experience. I had been through a lot already, but this, this was something else. And the worst part? The tube was now a part of me for the time being. I couldn't just rip it out and carry on, no matter how much I wanted to; I knew I just had to live with it.

The nurse used a syringe to check if the tube was in the right place. She attached it to the end of the tube and drew back a small amount of stomach fluid, confirmation that it had reached my stomach and not my lung. This helped me to breathe a sigh of relief after the traumatising past few minutes. If anyone out there has the option to get a feeding tube, don't do it. Dad later told me that during his nursing course, students had to give feeding tubes to one another, which he described as torture.

I couldn't honestly think of anything worse. But at least after all that, I now no longer had to stress anymore about trying to eat and keep food down. That made me feel a little less anxious, but having that tube in my nose was awful. I also felt even more trapped, as there was another cord now that I had to take with me whenever I tried to get up and walk around. Although I didn't walk around at all, just the feeling of being trapped was incredibly miserable.

I was glad that the previous treatments were all over, and now we could finally get to my last chemo session. I can't even quite remember which chemo it was that day; just the thought of it being the last one gave me such a big sense of relief. I felt empowered and like I could do anything, despite feeling so horrible.

I had a lot of mixed emotions when the last bag was put up. As much as I was excited, I couldn't help but shake the feeling that this wasn't the last time. I know it sounds weird, but it didn't feel real. After the first diagnosis and then the cancer recurring, I found it hard to believe everything that I was told. I was very sceptical, and I'm not sure if that came with me being older or my previous experience. It was hard as I had been told I was 'cured,' then eighteen months later it was all back. So I struggled with feelings of disappointment and confusion, not knowing how to move forward after such a hopeful moment like the chemo finishing.

In the afternoon, I found a tiny bit of energy, which was good. I felt glimpses of myself shining through, being talkative and trying to be funny. My mum came into the hospital on that day, and she even said, 'Angus greeted me.' I was confused because I am Angus, so I didn't know what she meant. It seemed like a weird comment to make, one of those things you might brush off in the midst of everything else going on. But later, after the haze had settled, I started to reflect on her words.

At that moment, my mum wasn't just talking about me physically acknowledging her presence. She was recognising something deeper, something that was slipping through the cracks of my illness. By saying that I 'greeted' her, she was telling me that I was showing signs of the person I was before everything, the 'pre-sick me'. She saw a glimpse of the person I once was – a little spark of who I had been – and it must've been a hopeful sign for her, even if I didn't realise it at the time. Your loved ones can tell when something's wrong, and I must not have been myself in the hospital. So, it was good to feel like myself again, even if only for a short time. It showed resilience and spirit, and no matter what was trying to bring me down, I wasn't going to let it. Even if for moments I let my mind win with the anxiety, I could get through this.

That was a small win for the day.

I also remember having a glimpse of myself for the first time so far on my phone camera to see what I looked like with the feeding tube in. Let's just say it wasn't a pretty sight. My colour was blending in with the white wall behind me, and even though I was sleeping so much, I still looked tired with big bags under my eyes. This was definitely not my best moment. If only my end-of-school musical had required a ghost for a role, I could have performed flawlessly, without even needing to act!

After a big day, I was exhausted and it was time for bed. No more chemo, and tomorrow was when I got my stem cells back.

I just had to keep moving forward.

Day 8

On Wednesday, September 9th 2015, my body was about to receive my stem cells for the first time. This is known as 'Transplant Day,' and it is one of the most important milestones in stem cell transplants.

It marks the infusion of new stem cells to rebuild the immune system. The transplant team referred to it as my 'second birthday', starting the journey to engraftment, recovery and potential remission or cure. This was pretty much the beginning of the healing phase, as by this point I had zero immunity, and when the stem cells were reintroduced, the new stem cells travelled to the bone marrow, settled in and would start multiplying. This is a process known as engraftment, which usually happened within ten to thirty days. The length that I would need to stay in the hospital was all based on this, so you want the engraftment to happen as quickly as possible; otherwise, you have to stay in isolation. After today, the team watched my blood very closely (as if they weren't already) to see how much had changed or if there was any change at all. It is very risky, because the chance of rejection is a possibility so you have to be monitored for that, as rejection is very dangerous and life-threatening. In summary, there was a lot to rely on today.

I hadn't eaten any food since Monday, and I was feeling quite ill. My blood pressure was low (no surprise there), so the nurses decided to use my feeding tube to feed me before the transplant was to take place. The food they put down the tube was quite disgusting; it had a weird yellow colour and resembled runny custard. Although the tube was still uncomfortable, it was a relief not to worry about eating and instead receive nutrition effortlessly. Another benefit was that I didn't taste the solution or anything else; the tube simply felt cold – that was all. Fortunately, I was just able to sit there and let my feeding tube do the job until the stem cells were ready to come in.

At around eleven a.m., as I was sitting listening to some music and chewing Hubba Bubba gum, we suddenly had a knock on the door and I looked outside. I could see a few nurses covered in the familiar protective gear that they always wore, but what was different was the fact that they were wheeling in a big trolley. Mum and I both knew what was in the trolley as they walked through the door. The nurses had this big, excited grin on their faces, and they pushed the special trolley right up to the side of my bed.

Suddenly, they pulled a bag out of a bucket on the trolley; apparently, it was minus 192 degrees Celsius. This bag contained 8,000,000 cells of mine that we'd harvested all the way back in May. It was quite surreal actually seeing them come out in a cloud of carbon dioxide from the cold. After the last week of chemo, it was nice to know that it was only up from here and this would be the start of the end. We just had to cross our fingers and hope for the best: that my body wouldn't reject the stem cells and the graft would work well. As the stem cells were my own, the risk of rejection was much lower, although it wasn't impossible, as the cells can cause weird reactions once defrosted.

We got the briefing from the nurses about what to expect, and they made sure I actually was Angus Cunningham (standard hospital procedures). Everything was normal until the nurses told me that the taste would be funny when I was receiving the cells. They informed me that the peculiar taste of the cells sometimes causes people to vomit. Apparently, patients described the taste as metallic or occasionally as prawn-like. Let me tell you right now, after not eating for multiple days on end, the last thing I wanted to be tasting was off seafood. I was already vomiting most days; I didn't know if I could hold it in if that taste entered my mouth. Luckily, I had the grape Hubba Bubba that I had been chewing all morning, so I was hopeful that all was going to be okay, and I could avoid vomiting during the procedure...

It was time, and my anxiety was off the charts. The nurses attached the stem cells to an IV bag and set me up to receive them. They were a weird red-yellowish colour; it was quite sickening to see. It was abnormal, unnatural even, and the sight of it made my stomach turn. It was hard to believe that this odd-looking substance was about to be infused into my body. Especially considering these were harvested from me.

As I've mentioned earlier, every time I had a new medication or anything really, I got anxious and stressed about having an allergic reaction. This was no exception; I could feel my breathing quicken, and my throat tightened as if it were closing. I took deep breaths and tried to fight the symptoms, as I didn't want the nurses to stop. I knew how important today was. I just tried to focus on chewing my gum and not worry about the external stresses.

The stem cell infusion started, and I was holding my mum's hand. It was a rapid process, as the nurse used a syringe to push it through my central line. I remember the second the taste hit my mouth; they weren't kidding at all. The taste was horrific; it slowly took over the flavour of my grape Hubba Bubba, and it was very overpowering. If I had to describe it, the taste was like an off prawn: strange, salty and just wrong. That's the best way I can put it. I instantly felt as though I was going to throw up…

Fortunately, the unpleasant flavour didn't linger for long, so I wouldn't have to endure it for an extended period. However, during those ten seconds, it was truly disgusting. It was quite anticlimactic, like this was one of the biggest days of the whole transplant, and the whole process was over in ten minutes. For something that had been brought up throughout my whole treatment process, I couldn't really believe it. It felt so unreal, but it was all done. That was it; now it was the waiting phase. These next few weeks were going to be horrific, as if this first week hadn't already been. The nurses briefed us on how, as much as I thought this was rock bottom, the next few coming days were going to get worse.

WORSE, I thought to myself. *How could it possibly get worse?* I already resented the feeding tube, and I hadn't eaten or drank in days. Apparently, the full effects of the chemo hadn't quite hit me yet, nor had the reality that my body now had zero immunity. It was like standing on the edge of a cliff, knowing the fall was coming but not feeling the drop just yet. As much as I felt I had fallen off the cliff, I wasn't even close. If there was one positive aspect to remember from this experience, it's that on September 9th 2016, I would be requesting a nice dinner and a gift. By requesting, I believe the correct word is demanding! I would be demanding a gift (only kidding… sort of) Although I didn't feel like eating, the idea of being free and going out for dinner was nice. It would all be good; I just had to get through this.

Worse Before Better

Day 9

The nurses were spot-on. I was terribly ill all throughout the night, vomiting everywhere. Even after managing to get some sleep, I woke up in the morning still feeling just as bad, extremely nauseous and unwell. I was vomiting up all the feeding tube food that I had been given throughout the past few days, so I did actually end up tasting the 'custard-looking formula', and let's just say it wasn't pleasant at all. I could only really stomach water, if that; it was more just to wash out my mouth from all the vomit. As my vomit was toxic, it was leaving blisters all inside my mouth, so I was in extreme amounts of pain throughout the whole process. This was my worst day so far as I felt so sick. This brought the anxiety with it, of course, which made me feel even worse.

Considering everything, though, the transplant team of oncologists, when they visited, were really happy with how I was going. They exclaimed how 'this was all normal and expected' and that I 'would get worse before I got better.' This was good news, I guess, and it made me feel a little bit less anxious.

After all the shenanigans from the night before, I then went to sleep shortly after the transplant team left. Mum said I was asleep for around five hours that day, which was becoming a common theme throughout these days. I felt so unwell while I was awake that I decided to just sleep. I did wake up, though, just in time to watch the latest *The Bachelor* episode with Mum. I know – such an educational television programme to watch while I'm in the hospital. It made me forget about what was going on around me, though, so I guess that was a bonus.

After *The Bachelor* finished, Mum and the nurses helped change my bed, and I had a shower. This was to help minimise the risk of getting infections, and I had to always (try to) stay as clean as best I could. I took the last of my nausea medication, which I was hoping would deter any possibility of the previous night's efforts. I wasn't hopeful, but anything would help. Mum read out messages from everyone as I was going to sleep too, just reminding me to keep my head up and keep moving forward. As terrible as I felt, I could feel the love from everyone. If I couldn't keep going for me, I would do it for them…

My quote for this day, which Mum loves to remind me about: 'Every vomit gets me closer to home; every day is one day closer to the end.' This was my mindset; I am sure you can imagine the scenes that were underway.

Day 10

Similar to yesterday, I found myself in a situation that had become all too familiar: I was vomiting and feeling extremely sick. I had lost two kilograms since the start of the week. This doesn't sound like a large amount, but when you don't have much weight to lose, it is a considerable amount. As we thought, the transplant team wanted to pick up the amount of intravenous feed that I was receiving through my feeding tube. As much as I needed the food, my stomach was struggling to tolerate it, and anything that was in it I would vomit up.

I began to become more and more silent, which was a shock to everyone who knew me. Normally, I could talk underwater, but I was feeling so ill I just kept quiet as I didn't have much to say.

My spirits were very low, and Mum could sense it. Since she is such a caring person, she decided to print out photos of our memories and trips in an effort to lift my spirits while I was struggling. She pulled one from our recent trip to Japan at the start of the year, which was my favourite. It was one of me doing a jump on my snowboard. It added something different to the room, which changed the scenery a little bit and made it more appealing than the usual four white walls I was surrounded by.

Apart from that, all I did was sleep that day. Even though I had slept a lot the previous few days, I spent the majority of the next few days sleeping. Being asleep made it easier to cope both mentally and physically.

We were only two days after my stem cell transfusion; I still hoped those white cells would come soon.

Day 11

By this time, I think we all can tell how much I hated having the feeding tube. It was uncomfortable, and I could always feel it at the back of my throat. Just the thought of it would make me anxious.

On day eleven, a solution to this problem was found. Maybe not quite in the way you would think. The day started off the same as all others: feeling sick, unwell and fatigued. The transplant team was still happy with how I was travelling, which was good, although it didn't help how I felt.

My stomach, now being semi-full due to all the feeding tube action, was making me actually vomit. Before, I would either dry-retch or vomit up stomach acid (disgusting, I know), but now, since I had actual content in my stomach, it would all come out. My mucus had thickened and turned into mucous membranes due to the chemotherapy. This made swallowing a struggle, adding yet another challenge to the mix.

At around midday, the vomiting started picking up drastically, which was awful. Every time I would vomit or gag, I could feel the tube moving in my stomach, which would make me gag more. This vomiting frenzy was insane; I couldn't stop vomiting and I didn't know what to do.

Suddenly, as I gave one last big vomit, I felt something come up with it: my feeding tube.

Yes, you read that right; I had vomited up my feeding tube. It dangled from my mouth, still taped to my face, the other end still lodged in my nose. Panic surged through me as my eyes filled with tears. This was, without a doubt, one of the most uncomfortable sensations I had ever experienced. Mum was just as shocked as I was. Before I could even react, she had buzzed the nurses to come in and try to resolve this problem. I had vomit all over myself with this cord hanging out of my mouth. I was surprised to learn this was possible, as they had never told me, but here we were; it was real.

The nurses came to the scene and, luckily, had brought scissors with them. Despite how horrific it felt, the fix was surprisingly simple. A nurse took a pair of scissors and cut the long, dangling part of the tube still hanging from my mouth. Then she peeled away the tape securing the top of the tube to my nose. My breath hitched as I braced for the final part. With one smooth motion, she pulled the remaining section out. It was an awful sensation, but at least it was all over now.

In the end, I was genuinely grateful that the tube had disappeared. I couldn't get used to it, and all I could think about was the feeling of it scratching my throat. The thought of it being out alleviated my immense anxiety, which was a welcome relief. This was until the nurse dropped some news on me that shook me to the core. 'We will have to put it back in soon.' I couldn't believe it; my body had just proven its point that feeding tubes and me don't mix, and now I was going to have to go through the insertion of it again.

Heartbroken is the only word I felt at that moment. I didn't understand why I couldn't just receive nutrients intravenously through my central line. The nurses relayed that we needed to utilise all my lines for other things and that nutrition via your central line is not ideal, especially when you can just do it through a feeding tube. I understood what they were saying; however, it didn't stop me from pleading my case to not put it back in or at least wait for an update from the transplant team.

They agreed they would wait until the 'bosses' made their decision about what they would do, but they did warn me that chances were that I was going to have to get it again.

That would be future me's issue, I thought, but for now I was settled.

After all this excitement, it was time for my usual sleep. I didn't do much else apart from sleep for the rest of the day. My blood still had no signs of life – nothing to show any response from the stem cells. This was expected, as it took a few days. We were looking forward, though, to any signs of life, which meant a step closer to home.

Day 12

Day twelve was one of my worst wake-ups of the transplant so far. My mouth and stomach were in agony. I was really struggling with the pain, and it was causing me a great deal of distress. Whenever I felt unwell, I would get more anxious and feel as though something terrible was going wrong. There were no exceptions this morning, and I really felt the severity of the situation. My bloods were bottoming out as well; my blood pressure was also extremely low.

To make things worse, the nurses were right. When the transplant team came around and visited, they were extremely eager to get the feeding tube put back in. Due to the state of my mouth and gut pain, though, they said they would give me a day or two to let everything settle down before they attempted to get the tube back in. Which was good, I guess, but the pain I was in was terrible.

The thick mucus and saliva in my mouth felt like fire, overwhelming me. I would choke on the thickness of the mucus, which made drinking water even harder. I found that the best way to deal with it was to spit it out, as there was so much of it. Yes, it was very gross, but at the time that wasn't my concern. I did, however, feel awful for whoever had to clean it up, because it would've been so disgusting. I struggled a fair amount this day, with back pain also starting to seep in. I was fighting many wars at once while trying to manage to stay positive and keep the ball rolling. After many vomits and much pain, I eventually got to sleep. Although with everything going on, despite everything happening around me, I still managed to fall asleep, hoping that things would get better. I wasn't confident, but I was hopeful. I was hopeful that I could stay asleep.

Day 13

I woke at about three a.m. with the worst back pain. My sleep that night had been rough, and I could barely catch a wink between my mouth and back pain. The overnight nurses gave me some pain medication just to help me get back to sleep, but I think we all knew that I was going to need something stronger.

The overnight nurses filled in for the day shift nurses and were in agreement that I needed a stronger pain medication. They had to wait for a nine o'clock meeting with the transplant team.

In the meantime, though, I was really struggling.

This has been a recurring theme throughout the entire transplant process, and it's the only way to summarise it. I feel truly fortunate to have had a strong support system by my side during this experience. I even empathise with adult patients going through a transplant; they wouldn't be allowed to have a visitor by their side the whole time. I was lucky my mum or dad were always there with me, as I don't know what I would've done without them. I am also grateful for all the lovely and kind messages I received from my community. I just remember in the dark times they would help me keep going and keep fighting.

The team agreed, and soon, the nurses were setting up a morphine pump beside me. It was a small relief in the chaos, knowing that whenever the pain became unbearable, all I had to do was press a button. A small dose would be delivered straight into my system, taking the edge off, even if just for a little while. The thought was comforting, but at the same time, it was unsettling. I had reached a point where I needed morphine just to get through the day. Although I didn't know too much about morphine, I still realised how strong it was as a painkiller, and knowing that I had it on request was not good. My young mind just couldn't comprehend why I was in so much pain.

As terrible as morphine was, it helped me to stay asleep. This was honestly the best thing for me at the time. Feeling sick and down would cause me to freak out and feel like something terrible was going on.

At this point in time, it's probably good to mention that this was all considered a normal part of the process, just another brutal step in the journey. But even through the misery, I had to remind myself how much worse it could have been. I still had to thank my lucky stars that I didn't have donor cells, because if I had, this whole ordeal would have been even longer, even harder and even more uncertain.

Day 14

I was deteriorating rapidly, and nothing seemed to help. I felt very unsettled and couldn't seem to calm down my anxiety whenever I was awake. In saying that, I was asleep a lot. I woke up in the morning and took some morphine to ease the constant pain I was experiencing, which ultimately made me tired and caused me to sleep. My white blood cell count was still zero, with no signs of any changes, but on the team's visit, they were mentioning that any day now there would be an improvement, and the cells would start blossoming.

I would rest, only to wake up in pain, and then the anxiety would hit as I felt all these abnormal sensations coursing through my body. It was becoming a desperate cycle; one I couldn't escape. This day in particular, I think I almost gave Mum a heart attack, for probably the hundredth time by now.

Sleeping was the best thing for me, and it usually helped cause less grief for Mum or Dad when I was asleep, as I couldn't be anxious. This had worked well for the past few days, and nothing really exciting had happened.

Suddenly, I woke up from my nap with extreme chest pain. A sharp, stabbing sensation shot through my chest, and I couldn't breathe. Panic gripped me as I gasped for air, my heart pounding like it was being crushed from the inside. I cried out for Mum, my voice strained and desperate. She jumped out of her chair and called out to the nurses for help. My poor mum, she was yelling out to anyone, but yet no one came; she couldn't find any of the nurses for assistance. As I was sitting there gasping for air, Mum was trying her best to calm me down while simultaneously trying to find a nurse to assess what was going on, because at this point it could've quite literally been any form of dangerous complication.

For what felt like an eternity, I sat there gasping, my chest tight with pain as Mum's desperate calls for help finally reached someone. Nurses rushed into the room, their faces sharp with urgency, which allowed me to calm down a little as they scrambled to figure out what was happening.

One of them pressed an oxygen mask over my face. I tried, but every inhale felt like I wasn't getting anywhere, like a fish trying to breathe on land.

Another nurse wrapped a cuff around my arm, and I could feel my pulse thudding erratically. I felt like my heart was about to burst out of me. The nurse comforted me by reassuring me that everything would be alright, bolstering my trust in their abilities. However, they clarified that an ECG was necessary to rule out any potential issues and ensure my heart was functioning efficiently.

The nurse then left and shortly after returned with electrode patches to place all over my chest. As the test proceeded, a lingering fear gripped me, making me nervous. The pain I had just felt was all too real, too sharp, too overwhelming; I felt like something was seriously wrong. For those few minutes there I thought that was it. I was so caught up in the moment, I didn't even remember to look to my right and see Mum sitting there. She was shaking uncontrollably, her face pale like she had seen a ghost. A frightened gaze had overtaken her face, and at that moment, I realised what I had just put her through.

I remembered all the times she'd been upset, or I'd witnessed her cry because of this stupid disease. At that very moment when the ECG was getting performed, I decided that for once, instead of her having the brave face on, I would put it on. Still with my oxygen mask on, I gave her a smile and a thumbs-up, letting her know I was okay. Although I didn't feel okay and was uncertain about my future well-being, I felt selfish for burdening her with my struggles. I'd put her through hell so many times, so the last thing she needed was more stress and angst. Mum's an angel and deserves the world.

My ECG came back inconclusive – they didn't find anything wrong with my heart. The doctors believed the pain was caused by excessive, thick secretions pooling at the back of my throat, which made me feel like I was choking. The nurses thought I probably did choke a bit, which explained the whole incident and why there was such a panic. I took some more morphine after that experience, which helped calm me down and start to put me to sleep.

The morphine pump would not be available for much longer, so I attempted to alleviate some of the pain. However, I still had permission to use the morphine pump today, so I decided to do so. I slept from about two p.m. this day; it had drained everything out of Mum and me. I even woke up briefly to see her asleep, which was good. She deserved the rest. We were in the trenches, but the improvements were going to come soon. 'Good things come to those who wait,' and my god had we been patiently waiting…

Return of the White Blood Cells

Day 15

The pictures on my wall were growing every day, reminding me of friends, family and good times. The sickness continued on this day; no chest pain scares, but the pain in my mouth and stomach hadn't really subsided.

As they had the whole time, the transplant team reassured me that I was progressing as expected. They assured me that the odd pains and symptoms were just part of the process and a result of what my body was going through. Although this didn't help settle my stress levels, it helped Mum to relax a little bit, which I considered a win in my eyes.

I didn't speak much during this time, which was probably a relief to some, considering how much I usually talk. As I've said before, people often tell me that I have the ability to speak underwater. I'm the kind of person whose mood is obvious just by how I act, a fact I didn't even realise about myself at the time. If I'm talking a lot and being my usual self, then I'm feeling good. But if I'm quiet or barely speaking, it means I must be really unwell. Mum and Dad picked up on this pretty quickly, so they kept the family and friends updated accordingly.

There were still no signs of the white blood cells growing, but we were getting close, we were told. The arrival of white blood cells would mark a significant milestone, marking the moment when I would finally begin to feel better.

They also removed the morphine today in an effort to cut down on my painkillers. Staying on morphine for too long wasn't ideal, and they wanted to start weaning me off it. I spent most of the day resting, which was a relief; as it meant I didn't have to be awake to feel the pain.

However, when the afternoon came around, I did start having conversations with Mum about our holidays and my friends. This afternoon was the best I had felt the whole time during the transplant. Mum and I joked and discussed our plans after leaving the hospital. It was a nice change from vomiting all the time and feeling nauseous. I still didn't eat any food and struggled to drink water, but I felt that I was able to talk. There was a glimmer of hope that things were finally starting to turn. For once, I felt a sense of optimism about tomorrow; it was a welcome change from the relentless struggle.

Day 16

Today was probably my best wake-up of the whole stay so far. I woke up feeling a little more hopeful today, like maybe, just maybe, things were shifting. The pain was still there and the nausea hadn't disappeared, but there was a slight change in my mouth; it wasn't as raw as it had been. It was a small win, but a win nonetheless.

The nurses came in to draw my blood, and I'm sure you can imagine that we were eager to see the results. My mood was different; although I felt fatigued and tired, something was changing, and I began to feel like myself.

When the transplant team finally arrived a few hours later, I could tell that they were bringing some good news. A faint trace of white blood cells was spotted in my blood. That's right, after almost a week of zero white blood cells, they had finally shown up. I use the word 'finally' as if we had been waiting a long time, but the team indicated that these results were actually quite good. This tiny glimmer of progress was a great sign, as this was earlier than a lot of people expected. They said tomorrow we'd know for sure if the engraftment had started, but even to be in this position was amazing.

This news was wonderful, and for once, it made me feel proud of my body. For so long, I had been so confused about why everyone around me seemed to get through life without getting as sick as I did. I couldn't understand it. Why was my body so weak when everyone else was so healthy? I didn't know, but getting the news that my body was finally starting to work efficiently again was a nice change. It was the first time in a while that I felt like my body wasn't just failing me; it was actually doing what it was supposed to do.

Mum also noticed how my hair had started to grow back. Little hairs were beginning to protrude, which was crazy, as for so long I'd had no hair. This was short-lived, though, as it was just in time for it to start falling out again. Typical, right? But I couldn't help but smile at the thought. I wasn't going to jinx it, though. I wasn't going to get my hopes up too high. However, the notion that things could be improving brought a sense of relief.

Mum left today, and she said her goodbye. She was heading home to see my brothers and get some rest. Dad took over for the night shift. He always knew how to settle me – how to make me feel safe even when everything seemed so uncertain. Today had been a bit better, and for that, I was thankful. It was a small step, but I was finally feeling like I might just make it through this.

Day 17

Once again, there was another day of improvement. The team was really happy with how I was travelling, but they did inform us that we shouldn't get too used to me feeling good, as I could be okay one day and then crook the next. My blood apparently had even more white cells today, which meant that the engraftment was happening! We were all so excited, but not as excited as the team. As they mentioned yesterday, I began exhibiting signs of engraftment much earlier than anticipated. I was having daily improvements!

With all the commotion going on over the past few weeks, I had completely forgotten about the musical try-outs. Well, on this day, September 18 2015, all the roles came out for *Annie*. I was so excited, especially as I was starting to feel a little better and the end became more and more reachable.

I had no idea what roles were up and what I would get. I had to wait for Mum's arrival in the afternoon as she had received the list via email and desired to inform me in person. This could've gone two ways: either I'd be disappointed or extremely happy. It felt nice to worry about normal things again after spending so long stressed about something so serious. It made me feel like a kid again, something I hadn't been able to say in a long time.

I even felt up to playing the Starlight quiz in the afternoon, which had been awhile. It was awesome; I was starting to feel like myself again. There was even a prize of a miniature Lamborghini, which you best believe I had to get my hands on.

I continued to struggle with daily fatigue and slept a lot; however, when I was awake, my sickness became less of a factor. I hoped it would stay that way.

After a brief nap, I woke up to the surprise of Mum being back. I can still remember her huge glowing smile; she looked so excited. Dad had been updating her with how I was doing, and I think she was eager to come and see me.

Before she even had a chance to hug me, I was dying to know what role I got.

Rooster. I looked at her with a weird look. 'Who's Rooster?'

I don't know how familiar everyone is with *Annie* but to summarise Rooster, pretty much, he is a charming but deceitful conman who tries to steal the fortune of Annie's family.

Mum and Dad thought it was hilarious. 'You don't even need to act!' they exclaimed. Evidently, I perfectly suited the role. Who would have imagined that I could play the conman? I'm sure most people who know me weren't surprised.

I was very excited, though, as it was a main character role. My singing mustn't have been awful after all. Mum also brought with her the lines for the play that she picked up from school. My teachers had already highlighted my part for me. Mum also said that everyone from school was sending their love. It was a great day; what could top it off?

Remember how I mentioned the quiz had a prize of a Lamborghini? Mini, of course, but I ended up actually winning it and getting the prize. What a great day! Honestly, that day was really special; it turned out to be one of my best days in there. I was feeling a lot better and everything seemed to be going well. I believed that the challenging times had passed and everything would proceed smoothly until the end.

I shut my eyes that night full of confidence, ready to take on anything I was hit with.

So I thought.

Day 18

After the past few days, I was expecting a semi-pleasant wake-up. That is not how my day eighteen morning started, unfortunately. A gut bug had emerged, bringing with it fever, pain and huge amounts of vomit. This was my first infection during the transplant, so when the team visited, they wanted the nurses to be very wary. They didn't want my infection to worsen, so I was immediately put on antibiotics since I still had very little immune system to combat it.

The antibiotics were forceful, and I slept pretty much all day. However, when I was awake, Mum told me about something incredible. Our family friends, Kate and Cha, who were all the way in Japan, had done a special ceremony for my health. They had gone to a temple and arranged for a Goma, which is a wooden block with my name and age inscribed on it, to be burned in a sacred healing ritual performed by monks. The thought of it was extraordinary. While I was lying in a hospital bed, struggling through this, people across the world were thinking of me, hoping, praying and doing whatever they could to send strength my way. It meant more than I could put into words. Mum also reminded me of the widespread prayers and best wishes from my community and my grandma's church. It was a special feeling, and it made me reflect on how much support I had.

Even though I slept most of the day and it wasn't as good as yesterday, it was great to know everyone was thinking of me. I couldn't put into words how much it all helped then – the messages, everything!

Day 19

The stomach bug was overwhelming me. The symptoms had not eased at all, and I was feeling a bit down. After such a high yesterday from everyone's support, the struggle hit me, and it hit me hard. Even though receiving nutrition intravenously was a better option than a feeding tube, my days were running out. However, as the stomach bug was making me continually vomit, they couldn't put it in. Which was a positive out of this annoying situation.

My blood was still continuing to improve. As terrible as I felt, we were still reassured how well I was actually doing, considering people would still generally be waiting for an engraftment, and mine was already taking place.

My biggest struggle at this time was keeping down the oral medications I was prescribed. These were going to help me kill this bug off, but keeping the medicine down was a different story. You'd think they would just give me intravenous antibiotics, but no. Instead, I was hit with an ultimatum, either take them orally or have them through an IV but with a feeding tube put back in. Best believe, I tried my absolute hardest to stomach the medication. There was no way I was going through that nightmare again. Anything was better than another tube shoved up my nose.

I've always given 100 per cent to everything I do, so missing out on playing with my soccer and footy teams that year was tough. Even though I couldn't be on the field, I still showed up to support the soccer team every Saturday when I was well enough. I would constantly enquire about the team's progress, even while I was in the hospital. On day nineteen, September 20, I received the Junior Clubperson of the Year award. When Mum told me, I couldn't contain my excitement. I'd hated being on the sideline, but I knew that my team needed me there, so I'd done it. To be recognised for this was amazing, and I just want to give another shoutout to Cronulla Seagulls FC for making me feel special. I still remember the moment I found out I had won the award. For that brief moment, I wasn't thinking about how sick I felt; I was just proud.

Everyone in the outside world was doing their bit to keep my spirits up, and I appreciated it more than I could ever express. I just had to keep persevering and fulfilling my responsibilities. But for the time being, it was more rest.

Day 20

My bloods were drastically improving; they were actually doing quite well. However, my fever and nausea were still a huge problem, coupled with the stomach bug.

It had also been officially two weeks since I'd last had something to eat. My appetite was non-existent, and to get even close to going home, I needed to be eating and drinking at an almost normal rate.

Today, I felt really down; I just wanted to go home. The better I felt physically, the more aware I became of my surroundings, which made me worse mentally. I had been stuck in the same four-square, white-walled room for over two and a half weeks, and I was fed up.

We were getting close, but there was still a long way to go until I could go home. The situation got the best of me on this day, which was all a normal part of the process. I wasn't saying much; I was frustrated and sick of everything.

As much as I hated it, I would never quit. I just had to take it one day at a time. One foot in front of the other.

Day 21

When I woke up on day twenty-one, I noticed a little bit of improvement compared to the day before. I still felt ill and sick, but the fever had subsided. I was missing home a lot; however, being on social media was difficult for me. Seeing all my friends out having a good time was hard, and even speaking to them was difficult.

I felt really isolated, so as much as they wanted to reach out and make sure I was doing okay, I stayed distant. Purely out of the feeling that I was missing out. Photos and memories were nice, though, reminding me that this wasn't going to be permanent and I would be back with everyone soon.

My bloods were still improving at a solid rate. The transplant team relayed how well I was doing on a daily basis, and how I should be happy with how I was going. I mean, I was; I just wanted to go home. All year I had missed out on things with my mates; I had not even been able to have a proper shower. I just wanted everything done, and I was fed up. It probably made things worse that I didn't speak to my friends much, but at the time it was upsetting seeing them have a normal life whilst I was trapped in this room. To be honest, I didn't speak much at all. In that room I had lost myself. I was down and not talkative, which I know worried my parents a great deal. To get out of the hospital, though, I had to start to eat food. This was still my biggest problem, and until then there would be no leaving.

As the day went on, I kept myself busy with my lines for *Annie*, trying to push past the frustration of still being stuck in the room. A visit from my brother Henry did raise my spirits a little. It was good to see him, and we had a good time together. He always cheered me up.

The nausea and fatigue lingered, but at least I had something to focus on. By the evening, I was exhausted, both mentally and physically. I lay in bed that night, hoping that tomorrow would bring more progress, anything to get me one step closer to home.

Day 22

I had finally mostly recovered from the gut infection I'd had. My blood was coming up, and I seemed to be doing really well. I was still fatigued and not hungry whatsoever, but these were promising signs. Although everything was good, my mood wasn't at all. The isolation took a toll on me mentally, and I was struggling. When the only people I was seeing was either Mum, Dad, or nurses and doctors, I found it hard to keep my spirits up. Mum and Dad, whenever they were with me, tried their best but had little success.

The transplant team knew how much I hated being in there, and they tried to give me words of encouragement. They constantly reminded us of how well I was doing on their morning visits and how, by this time, many kids hadn't even grafted yet.

As much as they were trying to be nice, when you're down, it's challenging to see the positives in the situation. I just wanted to be at home, for everything to be normal. It had been over three weeks in the same room. It was honestly like torture, and the longer it went on, the more frustration it brought.

The sleeping was helping make the days go quicker, but I needed a morale boost just to get me over the last little bump. Little did I know what was in store for me.

Surprise!

The isolation and confined space had definitely gotten to me. I was rough; I was still fatigued, but the homesickness made everything feel so much worse. Being stuck in the same room for so long, seeing the same faces was really hard. Not that the people weren't lovely, it's just I had a life to live, and it wasn't in this hospital. I should have been a carefree kid, running around with my friends. Instead, I was in a hospital room in the biggest fight of my life, experiencing things that no one my age I knew had.

Everything had really sunk in, and I didn't know what to do; I felt trapped. I wasn't in the mood to speak either as I just felt so horrible. My mental health had dropped, making me feel quite down. This made me isolate myself even more, with friends trying to reach out, but I constantly would tell Mum to explain how I wasn't up to talking at the moment. I needed to break free from this vicious cycle. At the time, the last thing I wanted to do was speak to my friends, which was so not like me. I needed a morale boost; otherwise, the last push would've been impossible. If only I knew what this day would hold for me.

Unbeknownst to me, my close mates had been trying to organise a time to visit me. Although they weren't allowed in the room, they thought that just being outside and talking to me would've helped me, as Mum was keeping everyone updated with how I was going in the room.

The sad thing was, I didn't want any visitors. As terrible as I felt, the last thing I wanted was people around. However, I am so glad that Mum allowed the plan to take place.

So after school, Reid, Vaughan, Jarvis, Kai and Lachy all planned to surprise me outside my hospital room. They wanted to come and cheer me up, as they had heard what I was going through and how I was struggling. All of these boys had shaved their heads for me twice already, so it's not like they hadn't already done enough. Additionally, they had all attempted to visit me on separate occasions; however, as I mentioned earlier, I never felt up to having visitors. The hospital was a depressing place, and it was the last place I wanted people to come and see me in. I had always been the cheerful one, the one who kept things light. The thought of my friends seeing me like this made me uncomfortable, almost embarrassed.

Anyway, this particular day was probably the best day for them to come. Earlier that morning, I was told I had to get my feeding tube put back in. You can probably imagine how thrilled I was to hear that. I was already struggling, and this news just made everything feel even worse.

I was sitting around feeling sorry for myself (as you do) when Mum told me that I had a special visitor coming. Almost immediately, I told her that I didn't want anyone to come and see me. There had been plenty of sports stars who'd tried to visit me during the transplant, and I would always turn them down. It was a lovely gesture, but I just felt so crap that the last thing I wanted to do was talk to anyone. So, when Mum said someone wanted to visit me, you could imagine my response was the same.

A few minutes had passed, and I honestly had completely forgotten about this so-called special visitor. Suddenly, Mum told me to look up at the window. I had no idea why. What was there to see? Just the same empty hospital hallway with the occasional nurse passing by.

Before I could even react, a poster with the word 'SOON' was slapped onto the window. Then another saying, 'WAIT.' And another 'TO.' Behind them, I caught glimpses of half-grown, dodgy haircuts and familiar grins. It was the boys! Deadset, the last thing I expected.

I was in shock. First off, why were they holding posters? And second, it was the middle of a school day, so how were they even here? I couldn't believe they came. I was so caught up in the surprise that I almost forgot to keep reading the posters: 'HEAR,' 'YOU,' 'SING,' 'IN,' 'ANNIE.'

SOON WAIT TO SEE YOU SING IN ANNIE

I reckon there was a bit of a mishap with the posters, but hey, I appreciated the effort. My mum was behind me, crying, and I might have shed a few tears as well. They were all smiling and waving through the glass, but until they picked up the phone that connected to my room, there was no actual communication, just a lot of exaggerated gestures and confused looks. As soon as the phone was in their hands, though, the real surprise began.

You'll be shocked by what transpired next. The boys then proceeded to sing 'Tomorrow,' the *Annie* theme song. This was when the waterworks came; I was in tears. Partly from the dead average singing from the boys (just joking), but I can't stress how nice of a gesture it was. I'll never be able to thank the boys enough for their gesture that day. Nurses walking past and patients all were crying too; it was a moment I'll never forget.

They were even granted a special five minutes to come in and have a chat with me. Even though they had to stay at a distance and couldn't touch me, it was nice to have their presence there.

Once again, Reid, Vaughan, Jarvis, Kai, and Lachy, you boys are the best. I'll never be able to thank you enough for cheering me up when I needed it most. That being said, I do have one request… please, never sing again. I swear the glass in my room cracked a little. Probably explains why everyone was crying. To the boys' parents, you've raised some incredibly selfless kids, and it's clear the apple doesn't fall far from the tree.

After a quick chat, the boys had to leave. It was incredible how this small action made the difference. You couldn't wipe the smile off my face after they left; I was on such a high.

I did still have to get the feeding tube put in, which the nurse reminded me of when the boys left. I won't get into details of it again, but I'm sure you can imagine how I was.

This day, apart from the feeding tube, was the best day of my transplant. Whenever I struggled or felt down, I knew I had support close by, and that was all I needed.

Thanks, boys.

Day 24

I was still feeling the excitement from yesterday, and I had the impression that we were nearing the end of our journey. However, my chattiness had still not returned. With the feeding tube coming back, I felt as though I was choking every time I tried to talk, so I stayed silent.

All I had managed that day was a sip of water, 15 ml to be exact; that was the extent of my mission with eating and drinking. The oncologist had just briefed us on the familiar rule. To get home, I had to eat.

Dad was with me, and he tried a bit harder than Mum to get me to eat and drink. So 15 ml was better than nothing.

Pretty uneventful day, but the vomiting did slow down, which was a bonus. The end was near.

Day 25

The oncology team was thrilled with how I was tracking. Home time was now looking less like weeks away and more like days. This was very exciting, plus it had been around thirty-six hours since my last vomit. We were coming to the end; we just needed to start eating. Easier said than done.

Now I wish I could remember who exactly gave me this gift; unfortunately, I can't. However, to whomever it was, thank you. I unravelled a zombie shooting kit. What a fantastic idea it was. We set zombies up all around my room, and I got to shoot them throughout the day. The perfect distraction, I'll say. My aim was pretty excellent as well. I followed Mum's only rule – don't shoot her – ninety-nine per cent of the time.

After spending most of the day working on taking out zombies, I decided to read my *Annie* lines and rehearse them. Mum was excited that I was prepared; it was likely beneficial for me to keep my brain active after watching so many movies and TV shows. I didn't read the script for long, but I definitely felt fatigued after doing so.

Although things were looking good, my blood test results indicated that everything was pretty much normal. I drank around 30 ml of water, which wasn't much, but it was a decent start.

The team told me that I might be home this week, but this was all the motivation I needed. The final push was on!

Day 26

After experiencing so much excitement yesterday, this day brought with it a great deal of fatigue. The team informed us that they expected me to experience fatigue for months to come.

We were still on the up and improving daily, but this was a big rest day. I managed to stomach a little bit more water, but still no food. That was okay, though; anything that I could keep down was a win.

Not much excitement from today either, just lots of rest and sleeping. I could definitely feel the fatigue setting in. One more step closer, but. Let's go!

Day 27

The end was within arm's length. Today started off with a massive win. During their rounds, the head doctor of the transplant team informed us that my blood test results were so good today that you couldn't even tell I had undergone the transplant. This was amazing news; we were so excited. My blood had recovered so much quicker than anticipated. I remember thinking to myself that I had to try and set the record for the quickest stem cell transplant.

This was all the motivation I needed to pick up the *Annie* script again. This time I was determined to give it a big crack. I wanted to be ahead of schedule with the acting and impress everyone when I was back at school. Yes, that is correct; this day was one of the first days when school thoughts started coming back to me. I could already picture myself back in the classroom, and boy was I ready.

I even managed to drink 390 ml of water today! This effort was massive compared to the last few days. The nurses were even excited for me. Mum came in around two p.m. and told me that it was the first time she could remember me greeting her with a smile. She even said, 'Angus is coming back,' signifying how much better I was looking.

This bald, skinny, frail kid had overcome everything thrown at him, and I was determined to get to the finish line, even if I had to crawl there.

Day 28

There was not much difference from yesterday, except I did gain a little bit of a temperature. I needed plenty of rest to ensure that my body could fight off any potential illness.

The transplant team just wanted to see me being able to eat food before home chats began. I had stomached around the same amount of fluid as yesterday, which was another positive sign.

Not every day in the hospital was eventful, and today was one of those days. The hours blurred together, just the usual routine. Mum (or Dad) was always with me, resting or watching TV while the nurses came and went.

Although it was frustrating, being uneventful might have actually been a good thing. No surprises, no setbacks, just another step closer to getting out of here.

Let's hope this pesky fever went away.

Day 29

Today, I finally managed to eat real food. Yes, you read that right; for the first time in weeks, I actually ate.

Now, you might be wondering what the first thing I chose to eat was. Well, I started the morning off with a bag of lollies. Not exactly a five-star meal, but hey, food was food. In addition to my gourmet selection, I managed to get down a cheese stick, some Gatorade, a bit of frozen grape soda, a couple of chicken nuggets, some water, and even a quarter of an apple. It wasn't much, but compared to the last few weeks, it felt like a feast.

The best part? The doctors had started talking about discharge. We were now in the 'discharge work-up phase', which meant Mum had been getting trained on how to use the pump and give me my meds at home. If things kept going well, there was even talk of a trial discharge that weekend.

After everything, the idea of stepping outside those hospital walls, even for a little while, felt almost unreal. Fingers crossed.

Day 30
2 October 2015.

I woke up early today with the six a.m. nurse who was there to collect my blood. Today felt a little different from all the previous days; I couldn't pinpoint why, but I felt good.

Yesterday, the nursing staff was teaching Mum how to deliver the 'food' through the feeding tube. This was a positive sign, and with my proving over the last twenty-four hours that I could keep stuff in my stomach without vomiting, a case was to be made to let me go home. We just needed to convince the team that I could finish the rest of my isolation at my house.

Nine a.m. couldn't have come any sooner. I hadn't spoken much to the transplant team over the past month, but on day thirty, they were definitely going to hear a lot from me. It was time to plead my case.

The team walked in, and I greeted them with a big smile. I made sure that I sat upright and had plates of mostly finished food around me to portray that I had been eating. I had to make the best case possible to be eligible to go home.

I was very attentive to the conversation they were having with Mum and me. 'Bloods are looking very good' was mentioned a few times, which was promising. The nurse even came in to vouch for me and back up my statement that I had eaten the day before and that morning too.

I crossed both my fingers and toes.

The conversation felt like it was never going to end when suddenly they brought me into it. The basic questions came first: 'How are you feeling?' 'Any nausea?' The answer followed the usual routine. But then, at the end, something different. The question was one I had never heard before, and it took me by surprise.

'How would you feel about going home?'

My jaw fell. I couldn't believe it. After a month trapped in this little prison, fighting through every challenge thrown my way, I was finally allowed to go home. It didn't feel real.

I had to pinch myself.

Of course, there was a catch. My immunity was still absolutely shot. So the logistics were that I'd be in isolation for at least another twenty days, maybe even longer. No visitors, no stepping outside, no risks allowed whatsoever.

Mum, Dad and everyone at home would be working overtime to make sure I was safe. If even a single germ managed to infiltrate, I would quickly return to hospital.

But none of that mattered at the moment. I was going home, even if just for a day. After a month of staring at the same four white walls, that was enough to make me feel like I'd already won.

Mum and I both thanked the transplant team for their help over the last month. They were awesome, and so were the nurses. The nurses were always there for us in any situation, and they patiently tolerated all of my anxiety attacks, which must have been difficult for them. There are some lovely humans in this world.

We packed up our stuff and called Dad to tell him the news. He was almost as delighted as I was. It was very hard for both my parents to see me in the hospital in that condition, so I think they were just excited to have me back at home.

It felt quite weird watching Mum take down all the pictures and unpack my cupboard. As much as I hated the place, it had become my little home.

After everything was packed away, the nurses got my discharge report ready and unplugged me from all the machines. I still remember the first time I stood up after not having all those machines attached to me anymore. I felt so free. Well, as free as you can be in a boot.

I wish I had a grand story about how I leapt out of the room, but in reality that didn't happen. I was so weak that walking was hard, especially with the boot, so we got a wheelchair to take me out.

I couldn't help but glance back one last time in the room as I was being wheeled out. So much had happened within those four walls, mostly moments I never wanted to relive. But now I was leaving, I felt quite emotional, to be completely honest; seeing the outside world was mind-blowing.

I'll never forget the moment I was wheeled out of the hospital. The sky was a brilliant shade of blue, very different from the usual sterile white walls I'd been trapped behind. The trees swayed gently in the breeze, their leaves bright green, and the air smelled fresh. The day felt alive, and for the first time in a month, so did I.

I grabbed my phone out of my pocket and took a photo. I wanted to remember and cherish this moment for the rest of my life, and let's just say to this day I do.

Dad was waiting there for us, and he greeted me with a big hug before he helped me into the car.

I watched the hospital shrink in the distance as the car left the driveway; it was all over. So many things were going through my head. I closed my eyes, and the last image I saw was of that big hospital. The lovely people I had met over the past month I'd never forget. This chapter was coming to an end, and I was ready for it.

Noah, Darcy, Henry and my cat Eddie greeted me at the door upon my arrival home. There were many hugs, but after the day I'd had, I was exhausted and ready to just lie in bed.

As I was closing my eyes in bed, I couldn't stop thinking about the new chapter that I was about to begin. After a month behind those walls, countless hours were spent wondering what else I could've been doing if I wasn't sick. But despite everything – the pain, the setbacks, the moments where it felt like too much – I kept on going. I was still standing.

End of Isolation

The first day out of hospital isolation was pretty anticlimactic, to be honest, as I was still in isolation. However, in saying that, I was truly grateful to be home. We took the wheelchair home with us as walking was still an impossible task, so there weren't too many celebratory dances.

My eating increased slowly, but still I needed the feeding tube to fill in the gaps in nutrition that I wasn't getting. The plan was to be in isolation for another twenty days, with two visits to the hospital per week. This was to ensure that I was getting enough nutrition and to monitor my blood, etc. On my final day of isolation, which was set to be around the 21st of October, I would have my final PET and CT scans to make sure that I was cancer-free.

Up until that point, my focus was solely on rest and recovery, gradually returning to normalcy day by day. I had plenty of time to work on my *Annie* lines, which would allow me to be up to date with everything.

So, I got home on a Friday, and it only took two days for some drama to unfold. By now, I think we can all agree on how much I absolutely hated the feeding tube. Well, by Monday, it was gone. Yep, you read that right. Gone.

I was scheduled to go to the hospital on Monday, so perfect timing. But on Sunday night, we all enjoyed a lovely family dinner together. We cherished these moments, as it had been so long since we'd been able to have them.

However, I got caught up, and I believe that I overate a little bit. In my condition, just one or two bites too many could be the difference between keeping it down or throwing it all back up.

I got excited, I think, and ate just that bit too much. By the end of dinner, I started experiencing a familiar feeling of nausea. I knew the best place to be when I felt the nausea was lying down in my bed. The sweating shortly followed, and I felt quite ill. I yelled out to Mum, asking if she could grab me some ondansetron to ease the symptoms and hopefully stop me from vomiting.

Well, it turns out that I didn't seem to have it in time.

Before I could even react, I ended up vomiting my dinner straight up. Luckily, I had vomit bags piled up on my bedside table, as this wasn't a little vomit either; I'm talking about a gigantic vomit, where the bag was almost filled up (disgusting, right!) Since my vomit was still toxic, I made a strong effort to avoid spreading it everywhere.

However, although the vomit was the initial problem, it didn't take long for me to realise what had come up with it.

You wouldn't have guessed it, but my feeding tube was once again hanging out of my mouth. For the second time. This event was meant to be a rare occurrence, and here we were; it happened to me twice.

I yelled out for help as I sat in my bed with this thing hanging out of my mouth. Luckily, Dad, having been a nurse before, knew what to do in this situation. I just had to sit and wait for them to get upstairs so they could free me from this mess.

Soon, my parents arrived, and Dad ran to get scissors to cut the tube. Upon reflection, that situation had to be one of the most uncomfortable things to happen to me. I was just sitting there with all this tension on my nose and the back of my throat.

Fortunately, Dad cut me loose quickly, and I was freed from the dreadful feeding tube.

It was a bittersweet moment. Vomiting up the feeding tube can be quite frightening, and I would be lying if I didn't admit that I felt shaken up. However, in saying that, I realised that I no longer had a feeding tube. This was what I'd asked for! But I did also realise that me being home without it meant that I would need to increase my eating to make up for it; otherwise, it was going straight back in.

This was not going to happen again; I couldn't go through all of that again. I knew that it was either go hard or go home.

Either eat or get the feeding tube. I had failed once, but that wasn't going to happen again. The determination was real.

It was funny seeing the shock on Toby's face when I rocked up to C2West on the Monday without my feeding tube. I don't think he shared the same humour; he was more concerned. I was exactly right; I had to ensure I was eating a sustainable amount of calories, or else the feeding tube would get put back in.

Not only that, but I had to have a visit with a dietitian as well to try and make a plan to ensure I was eating.

There was a bonus to all of this, though. I think I'll make everyone jealous when I say that I could eat literally anything at this point. If I felt like it, I was allowed to eat it: chocolate, KFC, anything. How wonderful was that! I had to take advantage of the offer before it was too late, as soon enough I would be back to the green shakes and vegetables.

The next two weeks were a giant blur, with most of my days consisting of the same routine, including frequent hospital visits. I was doing well, however, as my food intake increased during that time period. Pies were an enormous help for that, as I constantly found myself craving them. We were lucky to have a fantastic bakery up the road, so getting them was quite easy. For everyone wondering, I avoided the feeding tube, which was a bonus. I also did get sent home schoolwork after about a week of being at home, so I was doing that. In a weird way, I was actually excited to do schoolwork. After the year I'd had, it felt refreshing to get back to something normal. Especially considering I had technically failed Year 6, which was a bummer, but hey, I wasn't going to have to repeat the year, so that was all good.

Mum and Dad also broke some semi-heartbreaking news to me during those weeks. During an appointment, they told me that they had been researching and speaking with Toby (without my knowledge) about putting me on my old pal brentuximab as a maintenance therapy. It had shown success in a few trials, and after the cancer came back once, I could understand why they were considering it. Fair enough. It broke them seeing me so unwell that past year.

Mum and Dad didn't want to take any risks with another relapse; they'd seen me go through it once, and especially after how sick I had been, they couldn't bear the thought of watching it happen again.

As I'm sure you guys can imagine, I wasn't so stoked on the idea. For starters, brentuximab made me have that 'unable to breathe' reaction that one day, which was one of the main reasons for my severe anxiety and PTSD. Also, I was so done with all the chemotherapies; I just wanted to be a normal kid again. However, even though Mum and Dad said that 'we'd talk about it,' it was pretty much confirmed if I had a clear PET scan. At the moment I was furious and upset with this decision, but what could I do? It took me a few days to come to terms with it. Even the fact that I had to keep the stupid central line in was annoying; I just wanted it out. I hadn't swum or even had a simple shower all year. Mum and Dad changed the showerhead to a movable one for me, so I no longer had that excuse.

After everything, here we were, the night before what could be my final PET and CT scans. It was a situation I was all too familiar with. You'd think, after going through it so many times, it would get easier, that the nerves wouldn't hit as hard. I can confirm that was not the case. I remember being awake all night, feeling extremely worried. After everything I'd gone through, the thought of having to do it all again was terrifying. There was talk of another transplant if the scan wasn't clear, which was unsettling to even think about. I had already come to terms with having brentuximab afterwards, but a stem cell transplant? That was a whole different ball game. So many thoughts were flying through my brain that night, eager to begin the new chapter. I just needed the scan to be clear. Fingers crossed.

The day of the PET scan was October 20, 2015. I'd be lying to say that I wasn't nervous, but my parents were awesome that day. In a weird way, they sheltered me from my anxiety through the day. Anytime I had a negative thought about the scan and I told Mum and Dad, they reassured me that it would all be fine. They definitely felt the nerves too, but they hid it well just to make me feel okay. That's the type of people my parents are.

There was a tonne relying on this PET scan. I acknowledge that every scan is important, but to me this one was the most. After a clear PET now, I would be able to get back to everything. I would deal with the brentuximab when it came around, but for now I was just focused on getting through today.

The whole time during the scans, I felt my heart pounding in my chest; the nerves had definitely kicked in. I stayed as still as possible, counting the seconds in my head, willing it to be over. By now, I knew exactly when they'd slide me in, when the machine would start humming, and when they'd tell me it was all done. Each time, you'd think it would feel quicker, but it still felt like a lifetime in there.

Once it was finally over, I climbed off the table, stretched out my stiff limbs and took a deep breath. There was nothing else to do now but wait. Tomorrow, I'd be back here, except I'd be sitting in Toby's office, waiting to hear the news. Until then, it was the usual routine. Hot chips with chicken salt from the hospital cafeteria on the way out and then home time.

That night, once again, like I so often did, I lay awake thinking. Even now, I still am the worst sleeper; I just always seem to reflect on everything right before I go to bed. This night was strange, though. After the year I'd just had, it felt so long and like it would never end. Here I was at pretty much the end if all went well. Even though the brentuximab was still to come, which would prolong my central line coming out and still technically was chemo, that was it for potentially having cancer. I could just get on with my life. There was always going to be that distrust, though, as it already came back once, but still, like, what now?

I had pretty much forgotten what it was like to be a normal kid. I enjoyed not being poked and prodded every day, having no constant blood pressure checks, and avoiding temperature readings every few hours; instead, I could appreciate simple things like using a real toilet rather than those awful hospital pans (which were absolutely gross). I knew there would be an adjustment period; I just hoped it wasn't going to be too hard. I was a very adaptable kid, but even still, starting high school is never easy, especially after missing the previous year. Anyway, eventually after all this pondering, I got some necessary shut-eye, ready to take on the next day.

Wednesday October 21st, 2015
We wasted no time in the morning getting ready and heading into the hospital. I actually had two appointments that day; obviously the PET scan with Toby, and then I was also seeing the orthopaedic surgeon as well to check out my foot. Two big events in one day, one obviously a little more important than the other, but a big day nonetheless.

As I walked through the children's hospital doors, my mind kept drifting back to that day over two years ago when we first met Toby in the day consultation ward at the bottom of the hospital. Back then, we had no idea just how much our lives were about to change in the years to come. Now, here we were again, the three of us, back in the same place, full circle, but carrying the weight of everything we'd been through.

Mum and Dad seemed quieter than they had been the previous days. I think the seriousness of the situation was affecting everyone. I understood where they were coming from, but I was confident. Although of course I was a little bit anxious, as my body had been through hell and back and made it through the other side. I felt as though I could conquer anything, and this wasn't going to stop me. Granted, I still experienced frequent panic attacks and felt deeply shaken by everything I had experienced, but I preferred to cling to the classic line, 'What doesn't kill you makes you stronger.'

I will never forget waiting in C2North for Toby to come and grab us. Usually I would just pull out my phone and escape the outside world; however, I decided to speak with Mum and Dad. The topic of what we wanted to do when this was all over came up, and I couldn't help but mention the idea of a 'Japan trip' again. I know I was very fortunate to have been once, but another time won't kill you, will it?

Usually the wait was quite long, but before we even knew it, Toby stood in front of us with a big smile on his face. As I had mentioned many times before, you couldn't get too caught up in the smile; Toby always greeted us with one, but it didn't always mean good news. 'Hey maestro,' came the classic greeting Toby always dropped. Regardless of the circumstances, those words consistently brought me comfort.

We followed him to the usual room, the first on the left. You could've heard a pin drop with the silence that followed us as we walked through the room. Toby never liked to discuss anything unless we were in the consultation room.

After we all sat down, Toby decided to get straight into it. My heart was racing; I felt as though I was going to faint. I couldn't believe that this was the day. I finally was going to get the news I had been waiting for.

Toby said the words that I will never forget until the day I die. 'Your PET scan is clear; no signs of active cancer.'

It was one of the best days of my entire life.

I turned and looked at my parents; I could see the tears in their eyes. After a long struggle against this situation, we had finally reached our goal, overcoming everything that had been thrown our way. This was indeed one of the greatest moments of my entire life.

It also marked the conclusion of my isolation period. After forty-nine days of isolation, over thirty of which were in the hospital, I was free. I had my whole life ahead of me now. You couldn't wipe the smile off of my face.

That still to this day was the best appointment I've ever had with Toby. He did also drop all the side effects once again at the end. Most of them were the same old, but I would have to live a healthy life to ensure I reduced the risk of long-term effects. I had a much more heightened risk of secondary cancers further down in life, especially thyroid and skin cancer, coronary artery and heart disease, diabetes, etc. The list goes on. What was sad, though, was the fact that the chances of me having kids were unlikely.

Due to my age at the time, I was either just starting or about to start puberty, so things like my growth would be affected forever. This also meant that the treatment could have a significant impact on my future ability to have children. I may be infertile, but that would be a test I would have to do later on in life. Skipping past all the negative stuff, I was happy.

This was such a wonderful day, and I was so ready for what was to come next.

Toby also mentioned the brentuximab, and both he and my parents were very eager to start that treatment. Although I was not enthusiastic about undergoing more chemotherapy, I understood that the chances of a relapse after having already experienced one were still quite high, so to minimise that risk, I decided to endure it. They also assured me that they would closely monitor me to prevent any recurrence of the previous events. It was a big day of information and plans of what was to come next, but honestly, I didn't care. I was just so excited about the future.

Toby also gave me the green light to slowly start going back to school. Who would have imagined that a twelve-year-old boy would be beaming with joy at the prospect of going back to school? Honestly, I can't stress enough how wonderful that day was. The weight of everything lifted from my chest. I had made it through, battered and bruised mentally, no doubt, but ready to get my life back on track.

A few weeks later, the family and I were in Thredbo with the Steven Walters Children's Cancer Foundation for the snowy ride. The Steven Walter Children's Cancer Foundation Snowy Ride is an annual motorcycle event held in the Snowy Mountains, Australia, to raise funds for childhood cancer research. Established in memory of Steven Walter, who passed away from cancer at nineteen, the ride brings together thousands of volunteer motorcyclists for a scenic journey through the mountains. The event not only raises awareness and funds for cancer research but also provides support to affected families.

Let me just say what a wonderful weekend we had. My family and I had the opportunity to ride on the back of motorbikes, fly in a helicopter, try archery and ride Segways, just to name a few. The people behind the foundation were lovely and took care of all our needs during our time with them. This was the perfect way to celebrate the good news. It helped take all our minds off the dreadful year that had just happened and allowed us some time to get away from the stress of the hospital.

While we were away, Toby was behind the scenes dealing with the brentuximab, as by this stage it was agreed by all parties (except me) that I was going to have sixteen doses just to make sure that any active cancer left was killed. Even though I wasn't on board, I still thoroughly understood why I needed to get it. We didn't want another relapse, no way. The only thing I hated more than the brentuximab was honestly the stem cell transplant and the thought of another feeding tube, so I had to suck it up. Just lastly, I want to thank the Steven Walters Foundation for that weekend we had. I don't know if you remember us, but everyone there was lovely and so kind. My family and I had the best time, and we will never forget it!

After an awesome and inspiring weekend, it was back to reality for now. I was participating in half-day visits at school, as I wasn't quite up to full days yet. This was only going to be for a week or so, just to get me used to the routine. We were very busy working on the *Annie* play, so that was occupying most of my school days.

Everything was going smoothly (health-wise) with check-ups as well, except we had hit an unexpected hurdle with the brentuximab.

Hitting a Snag

While we were away, Toby had applied for brentuximab to be used as maintenance therapy for me. However, after we had returned, the pharmacy company had replied – and denied our request. I remember Mum and Dad being extremely upset and angry; we all felt a bit lost as well. As the brentuximab wasn't on the Pharmaceutical Benefits Scheme (PBS) list for my situation, we were going to have to fund the treatment ourselves. Pretty much if my cancer was non-Hodgkin, we would've been approved. A study published in June 2015 showed that it reduced the risk of recurrence in patients with recurrent Hodgkin lymphoma by fifty per cent, so we couldn't understand why they wouldn't cover it. This was our first taste of the inequality of healthcare, and it was quite upsetting. I couldn't understand it as a young child. When you're sick, aren't people supposed to help you to get better? Why would money have anything to do with it?

Now, you might be thinking to yourselves, what was the cost? Well, it wasn't just expensive; it was staggering. Each treatment cost more than $11,000. And in total? A jaw-dropping $187,000. Yes, you read that correctly: the total amount was a staggering $187,000. This is the kind of number that makes your stomach drop and leaves you wondering how anyone could possibly afford it. We also viewed it as an investment in my life. My parents were willing to do anything to get me this treatment, knowing how serious a cancer recurrence would be. My poor parents were even talking about taking out a payment from their mortgage to cover the bill.

I was as in shock as everyone when I found out about the bill. No person or family should be in a position where they have to crowdfund to save someone's life. Especially such an enormous amount of money. We couldn't believe it! Toby was straight onto it, though, and he had already reassured us that he'd applied for the Patient Access Scheme that would reduce the cost. He also reached out to some special people that he thought could help us with this. We felt completely lost. The fear of another relapse loomed over us, and the uncertainty of what to do next was overwhelming. All we wanted was to talk to someone, anyone, who understood what we were going through.

After about a week of back and forth with the pharmaceutical company, we still had yet to get approved for a drop in the price, and not much was happening. Toby was having meetings with them regularly, trying any way to see if the price could be dropped to a more reasonable amount, with little to no success.

I remember how anxious I was during this time as all the conversations we were having were quite scary. I didn't want to get sick again, and this drug was going to help prevent it. But we weren't able to get access to it. I just couldn't understand why.

We had met a psychologist on the Steven Walters Foundation trip, who lived locally, and around this time I booked in to start seeing him. He was the perfect candidate, as his son had gone through cancer before, so we felt as though he understood us and could help me work through my symptoms. I felt comfortable talking about it to someone who got it, as I would usually try to hide my panic attacks from most people, with only my close family and friends knowing. To everyone else, I would've just kept my smile and acted like nothing was wrong, as I understood from a young age that everyone has their own issues. I just didn't want to bother people. I also found it a bit embarrassing, to be completely honest, and I didn't want people knowing.

I was just so convinced my cancer was going to come back. After I'd gone through remission once, and then the cancer returned again, it caused me a tremendous amount of grief and trust issues. I was struggling to get through my days without multiple panic attacks. The fear was overwhelming; I just remember being so scared. There was extensive discussion about the possibility of a relapse and its high likelihood, as we desperately tried to convince the company that brentuximab was a necessity rather than a luxury. Also, to add to the difficulties with the pharmaceutical company happening in the background, it was all too much. It was a very stressful time for everyone involved.

After many attempts with the company, on the 26th of November 2015, we received a no. We still had to cover all the costs of the treatment. This was not good. We needed help, and we felt lost, with nowhere to go.

That is when we met some of the most selfless people we have ever encountered. Now, let me introduce you to the magnificent Kate and Richard Vines, the founders of a truly special foundation, Rare Cancers Australia (RCA).

Literally within a day of us getting denied for the brentuximab discount, Toby had reached out to Kate and Richard, and by that afternoon, they had already gotten into contact with us.

We were blown away by their dedication and unwavering commitment, which had given hope to so many families, and now they were going to help us. After her diagnosis in 1991, Kate, who is a rare cancer patient, found her experience of dealing with the disease to be very difficult. This experience ultimately led Kate and her partner Richard to start Rare Cancers Australia in 2012, aiming to advocate for better access to treatments, increase funding for rare cancer research, and support families, among many other important initiatives they undertake.

We had finally found the support we were after, and it was all thanks to RCA. After contacting us, they set up a portal on their website to help facilitate fundraising to raise money for the brentuximab treatments. Not only did they set up the page, but they also agreed to pay for my first dose to get things going. Honestly, they were so kind and supportive to us when we were in a dire situation, and honestly, we never will be able to thank them enough.

Not only did they do that, but they also got into contact with *A Current Affair* Australia to film my story and then air it on television. For those who don't know *A Current Affair*, it is an Australian television programme known for its investigative journalism and ability to shed light on current issues.

I couldn't believe it; I was going to be on TV! How crazy is that? We had gone from feeling lost and unheard to having enormous amounts of support and having steps to help pay for the brentuximab. All thanks to Kate, Richard and RCA.

Mum and Dad weren't as keen on the TV appearance as me, but Mum thought that it would be good to highlight the issue around drug accessibility and also possibly help with the crowdfunding. Both my parents are very proud, and throughout the whole treatment process, it was challenging for them to accept help or money from everyone. However, in this situation, that was what it had come to.

Once RCA got involved, the pharmaceutical company then decided to give us a discount on the brentuximab and take it down to $100,000. Funny how that works; I think it's safe to say that both Kate and Richard are very good negotiators!

The donations were pouring in from friends and from the community, which was heartwarming to see. Once again, as if they hadn't done enough, the community all donated some of their hard-earned money to help me pay for the treatment. It was truly a humbling experience, how kind everyone was to my family and me during this difficult time.

On Monday, the 30th of November 2015, we had a visit from the *A Current Affair* crew to film my episode. It was quite an experience, actually; none of us had any idea what to expect. The people who came over were all lovely and very professional. They showed us what they wanted to film, which included all of my family. We were asked some pretty hard questions, but we knew that exposure to rare cancers and the difficulty of receiving treatment were critical.

Many people across Australia are in a position where they cannot afford treatment, so it was important to raise awareness about this issue. In terms of everything, I was a lucky case; some people need to travel across the world to access treatments, which is mind-blowing. Kate even came over and featured on *A Current Affair* with us, which was tremendous for them as it was giving their brilliant foundation, Rare Cancers, the exposure they deserved. I hadn't watched much of *A Current Affair* before this, but I want to give a big thank you to the show. They didn't have to get involved at all, and they decided to, which was awesome of them.

We were told that it would be aired in a few days, and I was so excited that I told all my friends and everyone from school to watch it. I don't think Mum or Dad shared my excitement, to be honest. As I said earlier, I don't think they wanted to look like they were begging for money on live TV. This was just the situation we had been put in, though. They were thankful for the show, but it was just a difficult situation.

Little did we know what was to come from the episode. A few days after the filming, we got the message that my episode was going to air that night. As I said earlier, I couldn't contain my excitement to be on TV. I can't lie; I definitely would have preferred to be on TV for a different reason, but it was still humbling to share my experience. I told everyone at school that today was the day, and everyone said that they were all going to tune in.

There we were, my family and me, gathered in the TV room, anticipation hanging in the air as we counted down to seven p.m., eager to see what *A Current Affair* had crafted for the world to see. The nerves were extremely high; you could've heard a pin drop in our room. Before I was sick, my family was never really in the spotlight, and now we were going to be on an episode on national TV. All we could do was sit there hoping the episode was well received by viewers. Now it was time to see what *A Current Affair* had put together.

Wow. Those were the only words anyone in my family could say. It was funny at the start seeing yourself on TV, but it became very emotional for all of us. *A Current Affair* nailed it, and they did an excellent job of pushing the agenda. Kate also did very well speaking about the good things that RCA do. All in all, it was a very well-produced episode, and we were so thankful for *A Current Affair* giving us the opportunity. At the end of the show, they even mentioned the link to the crowdfunding page on the RCA website for my brentuximab.

I couldn't believe it. It was bizarre to see my name and my fight highlighted like that, knowing that so many more people outside the community were now aware of what we were going through. What struck me the most was seeing my appearance on screen. I knew I had become pale and lost weight during treatment, but witnessing it on television highlighted the extent of these changes. It was as if I could barely recognise myself.

After the episode aired, my family and I went to bed, each of us processing the experience in our own way. I felt a mix of gratitude for the support received and the sobering reality of seeing the physical toll the illness had taken on me. The broadcast served as a mirror, reflecting not just my struggle but also the resilience of everyone involved in my journey. We would have to find out in the morning to see how Australia took the episode.

I will never forget the morning after the show aired; it was insane! I checked my phone and saw hundreds of follow requests and messages on Instagram. People from all across Australia were reaching out, sending love, prayers and well wishes.

That's when it hit me. I wondered how the fundraiser was going. I checked the webpage, and I couldn't believe what I was seeing. There were tens of thousands of dollars in donations on the webpage; I couldn't believe it. Once again, people donating their hard-earned money to help my family and me out was unbelievably kind. The amount of nice comments and messages was extraordinary. Moments like this made me so proud to be Australian. It was a true display of kindness, generosity and the unwavering spirit of mateship that defines us on our island down under. We sure do know how to band together to help someone in need!

Australia saw a sick boy in need, and without hesitation, they rallied together to help. Even now, it still brings a tear to my eye.

In just about a week, we managed to raise over $220,000, far surpassing our humble target of $100,000. At the time of writing this book, that number ended up climbing to over $320,000!

The RCA website had even crashed at one point due to the overwhelming surge of support and donations flooding in. I still am in awe of the amazing people that helped my family and me pay for the treatment. With the excess $220,000, we were able to help treat other rare cancer patients in need. How awesome is that!

To anyone out there who donated, sent messages or supported my family and me in any way, I honestly owe you my life. There aren't enough words to express my gratitude for you incredible people. Your kindness, generosity and unwavering support gave me a second chance.

You are a big part of the reason I wanted to write this book, not only to share my story but also as a testament to the power of community, resilience and the incredible impact of human kindness. I'll never have the chance to personally thank everyone, but I will always be endlessly grateful for each one of you.

A huge thanks again to *A Current Affair*, we really couldn't have done it without you guys! Filming our story and giving us the platform to reach so many people made all the difference. You not only helped us raise awareness, but you also gave Rare Cancers Australia the exposure they so rightfully deserved. We will forever be grateful for your support.

To Kate, Richard and the entire RCA team, I owe you everything. Your unwavering dedication, compassion and relentless fight have made a world of difference in my life and the lives of so many others. You gave my family, myself and thousands of people across Australia hope when it felt like there was none, and for that, I will forever be grateful. Keep fighting the good fight. You are truly making an impact.

There are amazing people out there. They are truly, truly remarkable!

Rooster

Now, with all of this drama going on at the time, you would've thought that I had forgotten about my school musical, *Annie*. Well, you best believe that was not happening. Practising my lines was one of the few things that helped me forget the chaos of the past few weeks.

I still attended school during all of that, and during the whole process, it was still full steam ahead on the musical and the end-of-year celebrations. Most afternoons at school were dedicated to practising and rehearsing every aspect of the musical, including the lines, dances and even the costumes!

You could sense the excitement from everyone in my year as we were soon to be Year 6 graduates. Many kids were going to open days and were in talks with high schools. I was just in shock that I was in high school next year. As slow as the year had gone, I never could have imagined it would actually end. I can't describe how weird it all felt, almost like I had time-travelled this whole past year. As much as I had missed things, and it made me upset to think about, I knew that I had so many cool experiences coming up, which made me excited.

All that stood between me and Year 7 was the Year 6 formal and the school musical. After everything I had been through, getting up on stage and being part of something fun and creative felt like a perfect way to end the year.

On Tuesday, December 8th 2015, *Annie* was to take place. At last, it was the long-awaited day of the musical! I couldn't believe it was already here. Luckily, I had plenty of time to nail my lines, as I'd spent so much of the year stuck in the hospital with nothing else to do. To be completely honest, there weren't many nerves from me either. I don't know why; I just think I had a new outlook on life. The anxiety was still real, don't get me wrong, but things like getting up on stage didn't bother me too much.

If anything, I was more concerned about the change room situations. Since I had a lead role, I had to get changed a few times throughout the performance, which meant standing there in the change rooms with my central line hanging out of my chest. I felt embarrassed taking my shirt off in front of the other boys; it was just another reminder that I was different. But at the same time, I was determined not to let it hold me back. I had made it this far, and nothing was going to stop me from getting up on that stage.

We spent the day at the local high school in their hall, rehearsing and getting everything ready for the big show. I spoke to Mum about the change room situation; she convinced me to be proud of it and look at it as a badge of honour instead of being embarrassed of it.

She really is the best; that's all I needed, a few words of encouragement. As I expected, the boys in the change room asked a few questions about the cords coming out of my chest. They all knew by now what had taken place over the past year. However, not one was mean or rude about it; they were just curious. I appreciated their curiosity because it came from a place of genuine interest, not judgement. They asked questions, and I answered as best I could. There was no teasing, no awkwardness, just mates wanting and trying their best to understand. It was a small moment, but one that stuck with me. After everything, I realised that people weren't as focused on my scars or cords as I was. To them, I was still just me, and that's all I needed to go out and smash this musical.

The day couldn't have gone any faster, and before you knew it, the night had begun. I peeked through the curtains just before the show started to see who out of my family had made it. Grandma and Pop even came down from the Southern Highlands to see us perform. I couldn't contain my excitement; I was so ready to show my family what we had been working on.

Once we got our microphones put on (how cool), it was showtime. My first Rooster scene was much further down in the play, so my first time on stage was for the boys' dance scene. The second the music started, everything else faded away. For the first time in what felt like forever, I wasn't thinking about hospitals, scans or treatments; I was just a kid having fun. Let me just say it felt extraordinary!

The musical went off without a hitch! I nailed all my lines, and everyone absolutely smashed their performances. The energy was electric, and the whole cast brought their A-game. The crowd even got really involved and were laughing at all the jokes, which was brilliant. Some of the girls actually smashed the singing parts as well; it was wonderful.

Being the cheeky villain was so fun and enjoyable. I am not sure that I'll ever have a career in acting, but I gave it a red-hot shot. I remembered all my lines, which was good, and I felt that my jokes sat well with the audience. I guess all the practice helped!

Congratulations BBPS 2015 on the musical. Such a wonderful night, with memories I'll never forget.

At the end of the *Annie* play, I remember standing there with everyone clapping for our performance. I looked down and saw Mum and Dad with tears in their eyes. Suddenly, a few people stood up, which prompted a standing ovation. I couldn't help but just sit there and take it all in, with a huge smile from ear to ear. After the dreadful year I had endured, I found myself in front of my friends and family, having just completed the musical. I made it to the final curtain, standing tall, smiling and ready to take a bow. I will never forget that feeling as it was one of the happiest moments of my life.

I'd done it.

I couldn't have imagined a better way to conclude my junior schooling. To all my peers from Buraneer Bay, I know I don't see much of you guys anymore, but thank you. All of you made me feel loved and supported throughout this whole journey. A lot of you had your own stuff going on, yet still you all were nice to me and showed me love. You guys were a great cohort, and I wish you nothing but the best in your lives.

I received my first of sixteen brentuximab treatments on the 10th of December 2015, thanks to the incredible efforts of so many kind-hearted people from across Australia and even the world (so I've heard). As you can all imagine, I was incredibly anxious, but as per usual Dr Toby reassured me that it would all be fine. I trusted Toby, so if he said it would be fine, I believed him with all my heart.

Oh, how could I forget to thank Toby! I honestly don't even know where to start. You were there from day one, guiding my family and me through this absolute rollercoaster with your calm and steady presence. Honestly, all I can say is that you made everything feel just that little bit less scary.

If it weren't for you, I wouldn't be sitting here writing this.

So, from the bottom of my heart, thank you, Toby. You'll always have my gratitude. It's just a shame that you're a Manly supporter! I mean, we can't all be perfect, can we?

A New Set of Challenges

As much as I want my after-story to focus on the positive, the silver linings and the victories, the truth is, not everything was sunshine and rainbows once treatment ended. There were moments that were deeply challenging. The reality of what I'd been through didn't simply vanish when the chemo stopped. The after-effects lingered, weaving their way into my physical, mental and emotional health.

I wanted to believe that life would return to normal, that the most challenging phase had passed. But in many ways, a new set of challenges had only just begun. The road to recovery wasn't always straightforward, and I think it's important to be honest about that. While I cherish the positives and the strength I've gained, I also want to be transparent with everyone about the harder truths of what comes after. In saying that, my gratitude and appreciation for life will never change.

Anyway, let's get into what I got up to in the years following my treatment. Knowing me, I'm sure it wasn't too exciting... ;)

After a few successful brentuximab treatments, we ended up trialling the treatment through a cannula. This meant I could finally get my central line out, so there were no more plastic tubes hanging out of my chest! I could have proper showers again, go swimming and just enjoy being a normal kid.

There was a little bit of delay to that, as I actually ended up getting shingles and spent four more days in the hospital in late January 2016. That was very unpleasant; I felt like I was having a heart attack. I would strongly advise against getting shingles at all!

On Monday, February 8th 2016, a significant chapter in my life came to a close as my central line was finally removed. This moment was monumental for me; it symbolised the end of my battle with cancer. By then, my hair had grown back, blonde and curly, thanks to the chemo curls. The removal of that tube felt like the final nail in the coffin of my illness. Now, the only reminders of the wars I had fought were the scars on my neck and chest, along with the lingering anxiety and PTSD.

This was just in time for my Year 7 camp, which was a brilliant way to start high school. I did get an ear infection, though, which upon reflection wasn't surprising, as I hadn't swum in over a year! But camp was an awesome way to meet new mates and grow even closer with familiar faces.

I found high school difficult at the start; just the change was a weird concept to me. I missed primary school and my year a tonne. After everything we had all been through, we had become very close. Starting this new chapter was difficult without a lot of them. Even going straight into full days was tough, but just like last year, full days at school were scarce. Plus, all the missed school days due to hospital appointments, chemo and scans made the transition period even tougher. I would have panic attacks at school, and as helpful as the school was, it was difficult to explain to anyone how I was feeling. I continued on seeing a psychologist to try and help manage my panic attacks and anxiety. I found what helped me the most was distancing myself from the hospital and almost trying to forget what had happened to me. I wanted to just be normal and move on with my life. As I was still getting the brentuximab treatments, this was easier said than done for now.

I did get back to soccer for the 2016 season, though, which was very exciting. This was a great way to connect with old friends and to help bring my fitness back to old levels. It was going to be a challenge to get back to my prior fitness levels, but I was determined. I also scored a goal in my first game back!

On the 5th of April, I had another set of scans. This one, just like the first, was also clear. These were great signs moving forward. We still had enormous amounts of anxiety each time I had to have a scan, but seeing the negative results brought a wave of relief every time.

My thirteenth birthday was on the 22nd of April 2016. It was humbling to finally take a step back and reflect on the past year. I was so thankful to be alive and with my family and friends. What an unreal feeling. A year ago, everything had been uncertain. We had been drowning in unanswered questions, living day by day with no guarantee of what was ahead. But now, looking back, I could finally see it. The light at the end of the tunnel.

I also reflected on the people who had gotten me here. The doctors, nurses, my community, and all the amazing people who donated money. Thanks to them, I was able to enjoy another birthday, with plenty more to come.

The brentuximab treatments went quite well. I had no adverse reactions, and it went through the cannula smoothly, making the process much easier than I had expected. They were completed once every three weeks. Let me just say: those three weeks would come around so quickly. The only time I missed consecutive days of school was around the cooler months, like May, June and July. This was simply because I either got sick or felt tired after the treatments. My immune system was still trying to recover, so this was all expected.

On September 27th, we lost my little buddy Eddie. He was the best cat, and I will never forget him. When I couldn't walk or wasn't able to move, he would sit with me all day and watch TV with me. I was distraught when he died; it was a very sad day. I found comfort, though, in the fact that he was always going to be there with me.

October 19th 2016 was the last day of my brentuximab. The day was finally here. This was my final treatment. My last chemo. Ever. I lay in the bed, just like I had so many times before, but this time was different. This time, there was no 'next chemo session to book in', no more counting down treatments, no more cannulas, no more waiting in this room wondering what was next.

The moment the final drop of chemo flowed through my veins, a wave of relief washed over me. Then, as the nurse gently pulled the cannula from my arm, I exhaled the biggest breath of my life.

That was it. Done. Finished. No more. This was the last time I would ever have chemo, and that felt unbelievable. Of course, I had to get the clear PET scan, but things were looking good. From all of our visits, there had been no visible change in my neck, so we were all very positive things were going to be good.

My PET scan was booked for Friday, the 4th of November. As you can imagine, the nerves were running high. But by this point, we were seasoned professionals at this; we knew the drill, the waiting, the worrying. It didn't make it any easier, but at least we knew what to expect.

The last set of scans we had was all the way back in March, so this would be the last one for a while. Toby wanted to implement a new path forward if this scan was negative as well. After the brentuximab treatment was completed, the plan for moving forward became quite straightforward. A scan would be conducted after the initial treatment, followed by six-monthly scans for the first year, and then transitioning to yearly scans. After a few years, the scans would stop altogether, and I'd just have yearly checkups. This was because I had already hit my lifetime limit of radiation, meaning we had to be careful with how many scans I had moving forward. After years of continuous monitoring, I was transitioning to a more vigilant approach.

Mum got a call that night from Toby while she was out shopping. As she told me later, her heart sank the moment she saw the hospital's number flash on her phone. A call at seven p.m. on the same day as my scan? That couldn't be good.

However, it was the total opposite. Toby, being the legend he is, stayed back at the hospital to see the results of the scan. Two words, he said to Mum.

'All clear.'

Mum told me she dropped to the floor in tears in the middle of Woolworths. Poor Mum, that would've been a sight! Shoppers were minding their business and probably wondering what had just happened. But at that moment, nothing else mattered. We were free.

It was now over a year since I'd had a clear PET scan. The longer we went on without any signs of cancer, the more it felt real that we were finally in the clear. Now it was time to get on with my life.

In 2017, during Year 8, I decided to move to a new school, starting fresh in an entirely different environment. As I mentioned earlier, I found the transition to high school hard and I just needed a fresh start. My new school wasn't all sunshine and rainbows at the start either, and I found it a little challenging until I got settled and found a good bunch of schoolmates, most of whom I still hang out with to this day.

My brother Noah and I were also doing lots of YouTube around this time together. I ended up getting to around 900 subscribers before I stopped. We had the best time filming, editing and doing crazy stunts we had seen online together. I loved it!

The hospital appointments began to be less and less common, and the stress of the past years slowly faded away. I eventually ended up stopping seeing my psychologist as things had started to calm down. For a period, the less I was around the hospital, the better I felt. I still had the PTSD and anxiety, but the panic attacks had slowed down for a while.

In 2018, Year 9 turned out to be one of my favourite years. I eventually made my return to rugby league, joining a local footy club and getting back into the game I loved. We made a team with the boys from school, and it was exciting to be back. After a few years of soccer, it was enjoyable to play football again. I had a wonderful group of mates, and I was starting to really settle into my school. I am still mates with most of the boys from that time.

As fun as it was to be back, it was a tough season. After my mate Carter scored the winning field goal to make our first game 17–16, we carried on like we had won the grand final. We thought that this was going to be the beginning of a special year. Only to lose to every team and come dead last. However, despite the losses, it was a great season. This was the first year when I felt like a normal kid my age, enjoying typical activities.

2019, Year 10, however, was a really difficult year for me. It was a year filled with challenges, both mentally and emotionally, and I struggled more than I ever had before. Mentally, I wrestled the most internally during this time. After everything I had been through, I expected that things would start to feel easier; however, I found myself struggling with thoughts and emotions that I didn't fully understand. It was like the weight of everything finally caught up with me. I played footy again this year, but I had lost my confidence. I found myself having panic attacks all the time again, just like I had previously. Once again, I felt as though I had no control of my life.

I struggled and felt really alone. My friends didn't really understand what was going on, and I didn't know how to open up to them. The constant fear of my past had come back to haunt me. After I got better and stopped seeing the psychologist, I think I just let everything build up inside. I persevered, striving to progress, but in Year 10, everything finally caught up with me. I broke. My school was incredibly supportive, with many teachers going out of their way to help me whenever I had a panic attack. Their kindness and understanding made a tough year a little more manageable. I just constantly felt like I was going to die or something awful was going to happen to me.

I was super embarrassed of it as well, as at that age you were just trying to fit in and seem strong in front of your mates. Whenever I experienced panic attacks, which occurred multiple times a day at one point, I would sneak away to break down and call Mum.

My parents were awesome during this time and would answer the phone whenever I called and talk me out of it. For about a year straight, I would have multiple panic attacks a day and just feel completely out of it. I never understood why this happened to me, and I used to get really down.

To outside people, you wouldn't have been able to even tell anything was wrong, but I battled immensely. I hid from my past as well; as much as everyone knew about it, I only ever spoke to Mum, Dad or the psychologist about it.

We eventually ended up seeing another psychologist who diagnosed me with PTSD, anxiety and panic disorder. I would have multiple panic attacks a day and found life challenging to navigate. Everything felt overwhelming, like I was constantly stuck in my head with no way out. The smallest things would set me off, and I didn't know how to cope. It was exhausting, and for a long time, I felt like I was barely holding on.

I remember once at footy training I cried in front of my whole team as I had a massive panic attack. I'll never forget how embarrassed and ashamed I felt. However, the boys and my team were so understanding. Most of the boys and my team members messaged me afterwards to express their hope that I was doing well. It was a challenging time, but yet again, the support was always there.

That year was also the Year 10 snow trip, which I was looking forward to a great amount, as I missed it in Year 6. This was during my peak anxiety, so my parents and I were worried about sending me; however, it ended up being the best decision ever. I found that in sports where you have to be present, like snowboarding, it allowed me to take my mind off everything and focus on the task at hand. This trip was definitely a significant factor in my journey to feeling like myself again. Being out in the snow, surrounded by my mates, and fully immersed in something that required my complete attention was precisely what I needed. It was a break from the noise in my head, a moment where nothing else mattered except carving through the slopes. Looking back, I truly believe this trip played a giant role in helping me move forward.

Footy was also beneficial for me, although that year I suffered a few injuries, such as another broken foot, and a concussion. It definitely wasn't my greatest year of footy, and I found myself on the bench more than playing. We did do well as a team, though, and made it to the grand final, only to lose to our arch-rivals, the Joeys.

In my group, only Cayden and I remained at school. I'd pick him up most mornings, and those drives were some of the best laughs we've ever had. Most of my mates were leaving at the end of Year 10 to start trades, a big step towards their futures. They were excited to get out into the real world, learning on the job and earning their own money. I was staying at school because I always wanted to go to university. In our senior years, we had the opportunity to choose our subjects; I decided on math, English, PDHPE, modern history and geography, totalling twelve units.

After the tough year that was 2019, I was eager for a fresh start in 2020. However, the end of 2019 brought with it something none of us could have predicted: Covid-19.

An Odd Year

Year 11 in 2020 started off very odd. In the early months, we heard whispers about a virus that eventually turned into a pandemic. I grappled with self-doubt during this time as, once again, I felt isolated. But in saying that, so did everyone else. Fortnite with my mates became our way of staying connected, and in a weird way, we all got through it together virtually.

My good mate Kody helped me to feel the connection that Covid stripped from so many of us by non-stop ringing me and all the boys from school every day. He was everyone's glue – the one who kept the group tight, reminded us we weren't alone, and somehow made the distance feel less distant.

I tend to blur my Covid years together because it was such a strange time; I can hardly differentiate those school years. Numerous times during both years, we found ourselves confined indoors, unable to attend classes. I can't emphasise enough how unsettling it was to spend my senior year in isolation.

Aside from everything going on with the pandemic, I didn't want to let it get in my way. The year 2020, funnily enough, with everything going on, was the year I found myself. Despite the chaos and uncertainty, I began to figure everything out. The panic attacks became less common, and I stopped having nightmares as much. I began to find my peace, and let's just say I was ready to take on my life. My mates were also very supportive as well. If I ever needed anything, they were just a phone call away. I found it easier to open up and tell them any issues that I may be feeling. They also found solace in this, as everyone had their own problems that they wanted to share. It was nice to be in a group where you could be open about how you were feeling.

I became really close with my friends Lachy C and Carter, who went to a different school. We trained together in a group of three and were inseparable, since we were all still studying, unlike my other mates who were off pursuing trades. Some of my best memories from my late teens are with those boys. They weren't just training partners – they were my brothers, the kind of mates who turned everyday routines into memories I'll hang onto for life.

At the start of Year 11, I became close with a girl from school, and we ended up liking each other and dating through Years 11 and 12. Having someone who I could talk to about anything really helped take my mind off the past. While things didn't work out, and I was sad for a while afterwards, it was still a big part of my recovery journey. I'm grateful for the opportunity to be brought into someone else's world. It was an awesome experience, and I still reflect on those moments with a smile. Her family was also lovely to me as well, and I hope nothing but the best for all of them.

On April 22nd 2021, I turned eighteen. Absurd was the only word to capture the feeling, a mix of disbelief and wonder as time seemed to accelerate in a blur. By then, it had been just shy of five years since my last clear PET scan, a milestone that felt both distant and monumental. My family and girlfriend at the time joined me at a local restaurant to celebrate, marking not just a birthday but a milestone in my journey. I had officially made it to adulthood.

That night felt special in every sense. At the time, I believed I understood everything, but now, in retrospect, I realise how much more I still needed to learn. I shared a few legal beers with Henry, and we had a great night. After a childhood riddled with uncertainties and doubts, reaching adulthood felt nothing short of miraculous.

School was very weird for my senior year due to Covid, but I knew I had a job to do. I was always a kid who tried hard in school, but for Years 11 and 12, I wanted to get the best end-of-year mark possible. I set my goal at 90, and I was going to try anything to get there. My mindset was that I may have had to sacrifice a few parties and stuff, but it would all be worth it at the end. I had schoolies (end-of-year celebration) to look forward to, so I thought I would push myself and then reap the benefits at the end of school. I put my head down and worked. I tried my best in every assignment or test that was put in front of me. Don't get me wrong, I still enjoyed all the eighteenths and parties that being in Year 12 brought, but I was very conscious of doing well. I had a good balance, and as I said, despite the craziness of the world at the time, I had a great year.

I finished Year 12 with an ATAR of 89.40, just shy of the 90 I had aimed for. It stung a little at first, but looking back, I was proud of what I had achieved. After everything I had been through, making it to the finish line and doing well was a victory in itself.

I just want to give a giant shoutout to my school, Cronulla High. The teachers there, along with the principal, Mr Ibrahim, and the deputy at the time, Mr Burnett, were incredible during Covid. Despite all the challenges, lockdowns, social distancing and uncertainty, they went above and beyond to make our Year 12 experience as special as possible. I'll always be grateful for their support and effort during such a tough time. Mrs Ward, my PDHPE teacher, and my mentor, Mr Kelly, always pushed and believed in me, and for that I will never forget it.

Thank you to everyone from Cronulla High; I need to come and visit some time!

I decided to go to the University of Technology, Sydney (UTS). There I was, going to study a double degree that included a Bachelor of Business and Bachelor of Creative Intelligence and Innovation. Not many kids from my school were going there, so it was going to be a completely fresh start.

My school year ended up going to Byron Bay for a week in December 2021 for our end-of-year celebrations. It was a fantastic week; however, on Day 3, we ended up having a Covid outbreak and a heap of kids ended up contracting the disease. By Day 5, kids were flying home and rooms were being isolated. Quite satirical when you think about it, how to top the year off, Covid had to make its way to our end-of-school celebrations.

A few weeks after we got home from Schoolies, I came down with Covid, but not quite how I expected. We were heading off on a family trip down the South Coast, and I was driving there with my brothers. I had just been at a music festival on New Year's Eve and felt unwell, but I didn't think much of it.

The day after we arrived, after a four-hour drive down the coast, I officially tested positive. That meant I had to leave, so Dad drove me two and a half hours back (with a mask on and the windows all down) to drop me off with my mate Carter, who had kindly driven down to pick me up. Conveniently, he also had Covid, so we figured we'd just isolate together at my place for the week since no one else was home.

We had an incredible week. We lived off steak and watched the entire Test cricket series between Australia and England. It wasn't exactly how I imagined starting the new year, but in a strange way, it was one of the best weeks ever. It definitely set the tone for the year.

Just a few weeks later, February rolled around and brought my first proper trip away as an adult – a boys' weekend to the Gold Coast with Carter and Kurtis. Kurtis brought the energy and laughs, the perfect bloke to match Carter and me stride for stride. He slotted in effortlessly, and together we made the most of every moment. We were fresh eighteen year olds, wide-eyed and navigating the big world for the first time on our own. What a fabulous weekend it was – full of laughs, lessons and the kind of memories you never forget.

The year 2022 became one of celebration with my mates, but also one of deep reflection. I found myself missing high school more than I ever expected. I was lucky to have been part of such a wonderful cohort. Saying goodbye wasn't easy. But I knew I needed to embrace the freedom and challenges that came with adulthood. I saw less and less of the kids from school, but I hope they're all out there carving their own paths and enjoying themselves.

I lived at my friend Kauan's apartment for a few weeks early in the year. Sometimes things were tough after first leaving school, just dealing with the change. He offered for me to stay with him and chat, which was precisely what I needed at the time. Thanks again, mate, for always being there for me!

My family, Mum's friend Paula, my brother Henry's girlfriend Mya, and I embarked on an unforgettable seven-day paddle adventure to Cairns. Cairns was absolutely stunning. We saw sharks, dolphins, stingrays and all sorts of amazing marine life.

My brothers and I got closer than ever without any technology to distract us. We spent an entire week camping on the beaches throughout Hinchinbrook Island, totally off the grid. It was pure joy, laughing around the campfire, paddling through crystal-clear waters and falling asleep under the stars to the sound of the ocean. Honestly, it was one of the best times of my life.

Quick shoutout to Mya for putting up with us. She's always been so patient with me and has never hesitated to give me her time for a chat. I honestly wouldn't want anyone else to be part of our family.

In the later months of 2022, I had the opportunity to attend the ten-year Rare Cancers Australia dinner, which was a wonderful night. After so long, I grew distant from RCA and that part of my life, and I had forgotten how important they were to me. This was just the way I dealt with my trauma from the past. While I was listening to the wonderful Kate Vines announce her retirement, I decided then and there that I wanted to help RCA like they had helped me. I spoke to Kate, Richard and a few RCA people after the dinner and put my name up to assist in any way I could.

Getting back in contact with Rare Cancers was one of the best decisions I ever made. It reminded me just how lucky I was to be alive and completely shifted my mindset. I'll be honest, I used to get caught up in things that really didn't matter. But reconnecting with that part of my life helped me stop running from it and start appreciating it for what it was.

After I got sick, all I wanted to do was move on and forget it ever happened. However, I realised that what had happened to me was actually a hidden blessing. It gave me perspective. It made me grateful, not just for life itself, but for the people who fought for me, stood by me and supported me through it all.

From that point on, I tried to live with a glass-half-full mindset. I knew what really mattered. I didn't take things for granted like I used to. And I was genuinely thankful for everything, both the good and the hard, because it had all shaped who I was.

A New Path

Supporting Rare Cancers led me to one of the greatest privileges I could've ever been given, an opportunity to speak at Parliament House for CanForum 2022. This was a rare privilege, an opportunity I'll always cherish. Henry and I went for the weekend, and it was the best time.

As I stepped onto the stage, my heart pounded in my chest. Speaking in front of strangers about my story was nerve-wracking, but knowing that it made a difference was a true honour. Although I did speak really fast and forgot to click my slide, I was proud of myself. Going from barely talking about my childhood sickness to sharing my story in front of strangers, and even people back home watching the livestream, was a huge moment for me. Having Henry there made it even more special. He was the perfect person to have by my side, supporting me every step of the way.

We had a great night afterwards, having a few beers with the RCA team. Henry and I then went around and explored Canberra.

At the end of 2022, I discovered my passion for running. For years, I had thoroughly enjoyed going to the gym; it had been a constant since I was sixteen. However, my dad, a former Ironman and competitive triathlete, persistently encouraged me to join him on his runs. His persistence paid off, and eventually I went for it and started. I loved it, and it became a new hobby that I was obsessed with. Running became an excellent way to clear my head and feel healthier.

In July 2023, my mate Lachy (who had shaved his head for me twice) and I decided to raise money for rare cancers. Lachy's dad, Andrew, was diagnosed with a rare cancer, and unfortunately, he passed away. He was a great man, and Lachy and I thought that it would be a terrific idea to raise some money for rare cancers in his honour.

After the inspiring act that Aaron Raper did with the Run 4 Angus back in 2015, we decided to once again take on the infamous Shire race, the 'Sutherland 2 Surf,' an eleven kilometre run from Sutherland to Cronulla, to support the cause. The supportive Shire community rallied behind us once again, helping us raise over $8,500 for Rare Cancers. We exceeded our goal of $5,000, which was amazing. It was an unforgettable day, with so many locals coming out to support us. We handed out Rare Cancers singlets, and together, we all took on the race. Mum and Dad also got people from their work involved, so people travelled all across Sydney to participate for us. Once again, the only word that I can think of is *honoured*.

The best part of our running fundraiser wasn't just crossing the finish line; it was seeing the impact Lachy and I had on others. Together, we managed to inspire people who were hesitant, even nervous, about running to join in. Most had little to no running experience, but they laced up and took on the challenge. Seeing everyone smile was also heart-warming.

Speaking of running, December 2023 brought one of the most unforgettable adventures yet: the Coast 2 Kosciuszko ultramarathon. My dad decided to take on this unbelievable challenge, which included a gruelling 240-kilometre run from the South Coast all the way to Mount Kosciuszko, the highest point in Australia. Yes, you read that correctly. Two hundred and forty kilometres! It was a feat so extraordinary it felt magical to witness.

Mum, Henry and I, along with a few of Dad's mates, were there to crew for him. Being part of the crew for a race like this isn't just a support role; it's an experience in itself. We kept him fed and hydrated, ran alongside him at different stretches and offered encouragement. Seeing him push his body and mind to the absolute limit was nothing short of inspiring. It wasn't easy, far from it, but the determination in his eyes and the drive in his steps made it clear how much this challenge meant to him. No matter how sore or fatigued he was, the last thing on his mind was quitting.

After thirty-eight gruelling hours, Dad crossed the finish line. Watching him achieve something so monumental was one of the proudest moments of my life. His resilience and mental strength throughout the race were inspiring, a reminder of what humans can accomplish with sheer determination. That adventure concluded on a high note, leaving me inspired by his resilience and drive.

Now, moving forward to a new chapter, 2024 was my best year yet. For my twenty-first birthday in April, my family, my mate Kody and I embarked on an adventure, flying down to Tasmania for a week. We stayed at Freycinet Bay, a place so magical it felt like stepping into a dream. We indulged in whisky tastings, savoured fresh lobsters, cruised along breathtaking waters, tackled scenic hikes, and enjoyed everything Tasmania had to offer. My family went all out to spoil me, and it made for the kind of birthday celebration that will stay with me forever. As my Pop so perfectly put it, 'The best twenty-first I've ever been to!' And honestly, he wasn't wrong. The entire celebration was nothing short of magical. I will never forget it.

Now, if I hadn't had enough travel for one year, I ended up travelling to Barcelona for university to do a global short programme in July. I was in Europe for six weeks, and it was one of the greatest times of my life. I mean, how could you go wrong with a Euro summer?

As a result, I now have friends all across the world, and I will always remember the experiences. I met two of my mates, Kobey and Matt, in certain places, along with a crew of Shire boys, and it was so much fun. We all had the best time travelling. Since the start of 2023, I have been studying Spanish.

Well, when I say studying, it's a very, very loose term, but I was giving it a crack. Matt and I went around speaking our terrible Spanish. We actually didn't do too badly from my perspective, of course, but it was the time of my life.

I loved meeting new people and just hearing about people's different experiences. I was also the token Aussie in the university course, which I thoroughly enjoyed. Some of my classmates had never met an Australian before either, so the conversations were always funny and exciting.

I arrived back home in early August, only to hop on board another flight two weeks later for one of my best mate's Kody's birthday. There were eleven of us flying to Bali for ten days, and we were all so excited. The first three days were so fun; we went out partying and just enjoyed the beauty of Bali. However, it didn't take long for disaster to strike and, funnily enough, it happened on Kody's actual birthday. My roommate in the villa, Matt, went down first with Bali belly, followed by a string of the boys. I was the fourth person to get sick. After a few visits from doctors, plus IVs and a few days of rest, the boys all seemed to come good, except me.

After feeling sick for the remainder of the trip, I was finally diagnosed with appendicitis when we flew back into Sydney. What followed was an unexpected five-day stay in the hospital. Despite the circumstances, I managed to find moments of good fun within the hospital. Yet, as lighthearted as some of the experience was, being back in there stirred some deep memories, both haunting and vivid, from earlier chapters of my life. Despite the haunting memories, I remained resilient and maintained a positive outlook. At the end of the day, it was a great story to tell. We will always remember it as the trip from hell, especially Dave, who got hit in the eye with his beer bottle cap. He had to fly home early, the poor guy. It took a few months to recover from everything, but I bounced back and was all good.

As I sit down to write this book, life feels brighter than ever. I'm working two days in the city and spending two days at uni, balancing both worlds while moving closer to finishing my Creative Intelligence and Innovation degree at the end of 2025. Having already completed my business degree, I feel proud of how far I've come academically.

What makes this moment even more special is that I'm coming up to my tenth year in remission. Reflecting on everything I've overcome to get here, it feels unbelievable and incredibly meaningful. This milestone is a testament to the people who have supported me through every step of this journey I've been on and the strength I've gained along the way.

Looking back on my journey, I'm reminded of all the wonderful people who have been part of it, some who remain close to me today, and others whose paths have diverged from mine over the years. Whether they're still in my life or not, I'll never forget the kindness, support and love they showed me. Each person played a part in helping me get to where I am now, and for that, I'll always be grateful. Their impact is a part of my story, and I carry it with me every single day.

Angus Cunningham

I completed my first marathon in February 2025 with my mates Luke and Zak. Truth be told, this was one of the most mentally challenging things I have ever done. Once I'd run thirty kilometres, I hit a huge wall, and every step became a cramp. I finished it, though, and I was absolutely over the moon. The sense of accomplishment after pushing through those final brutal kilometres was like nothing I've ever felt before. Sharing the experience with Luke and Zak made it all the better as we supported each other through the highs and lows. Completing that marathon taught me so much about tenacity and determination. It reminded me of how far I've come, both physically and mentally.

Recently, I returned from a seven-day hiking adventure along the Cradle Mountain trail with Dad and his mates. What a week it was, filled with laughs, camaraderie and amazing moments. The side tracks made it even more special, especially the climb up Mount Ossa, the highest peak in Tasmania. We had an absolute blast, and before the week was up, we were already talking about plans for more hikes in the future. We saw snakes, swam in cold rivers and sang 'Dancing on the Ceiling' by Lionel Richie. How much better could it get! I've been so lucky to embark on fantastic adventures, always surrounded by the most amazing people. It's a constant reminder of how fortunate I am, and I couldn't be more grateful.

Right now, I can confidently say I'm the happiest I've ever been. Truly. The older I get, the more I find myself appreciating life and recognising how blessed I am. These days, you'd be hard-pressed to wipe the smile off my face! I'm surrounded by the best friends anyone could ask for. Whether it's Jak faithfully upholding his weekly 'Angus Check-Up' or Emily sending a concerned message after a few days of radio silence, only to find out I simply forgot to mention I was off climbing mountains in Tasmania.

Although my anxiety and PTSD still show up on occasion, I've learned to handle them on my own most of the time by going on long runs, or talking through matters with my family and friends. I am so excited to see what the future holds.

Now, my final thanks. My family. You guys all made huge sacrifices to get me to where I am today; I just want to lastly give you an enormous 'thank you' from the bottom of my heart. Mum had to quit her dream job as a lawyer to help take care of me while I was sick. Dad had to miss hospital appointments and didn't get to stay with me as much as he would've liked due to work, and I know that was hard on you, but I understand. You guys were awesome, and I love you so much.

Henry, Noah and Darcy all struggled in their own ways when I was sick. I could never imagine what it would be like to see your own flesh and blood so unwell. They would've known everything that was going on and had to be brave and carry on. To you boys, I thank you. I know you did it tough, and I can't thank you all enough. I love you all, and I couldn't have asked for a better bunch of brothers.

Also, a quick shoutout to Grandma and Pop for practically living at our house while I was sick. You guys all are the real heroes, and I will always appreciate everything you did for me.

There are so many people that I haven't been able to mention in this book that I wish I could, and you know who you are. For everyone that's ever picked up my phone call, chatted with me, been there for me or even just smiled in the hallway at school or uni, thank you. I am so grateful for the people I have encountered in my life.

The things I experienced as a kid will stay with me forever, but through the support of my loved ones and even complete strangers, I'm still here today. Their kindness and generosity carried me through the darkest times, and for that, I'll always cherish you.

Though I've lived many lives in my short existence, this is just the beginning of my story. I was fortunate enough to be given another shot at life. Now let's see what I can do with it!

Thank you for reading my book. It's been an honour to share my story with you all.

Angus.

Photo Gallery

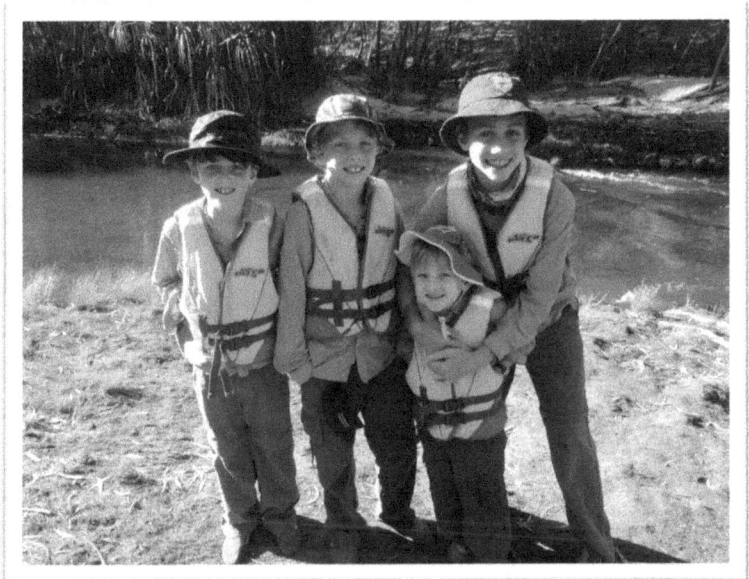

HAND: Henry, Angus, Noah, Darcy. With my three brothers.

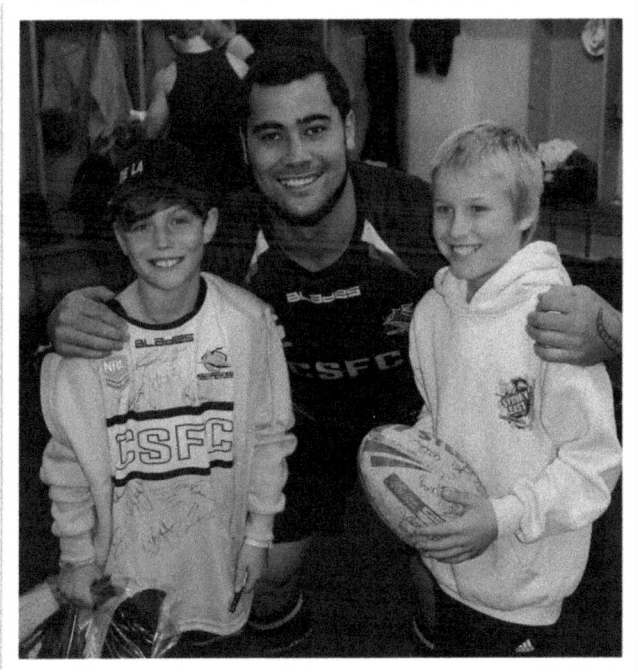

Kai and me with Andrew Fifita.

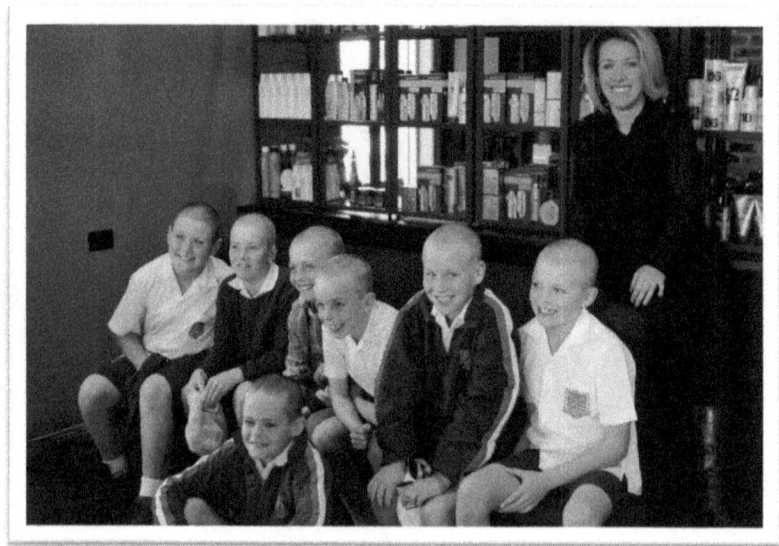

My mates shaving their heads with me in 2013.

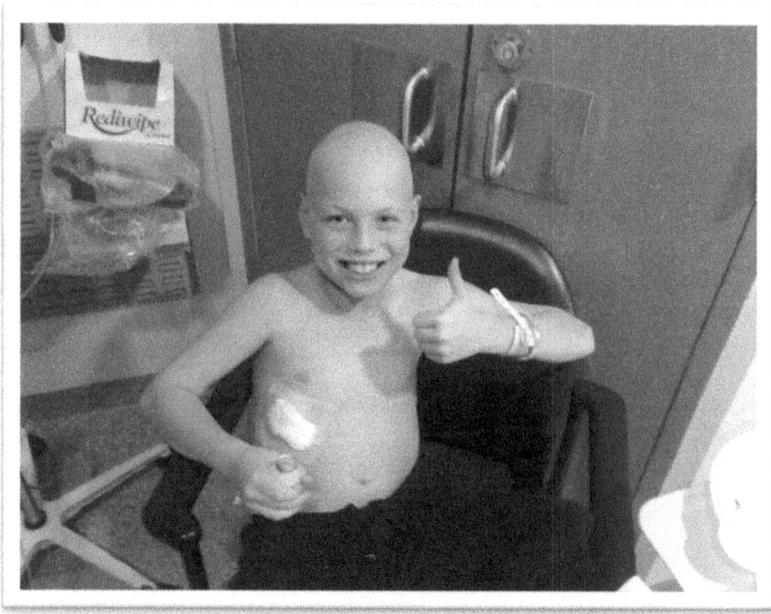

Hospital visit, trying my best to stay positive.

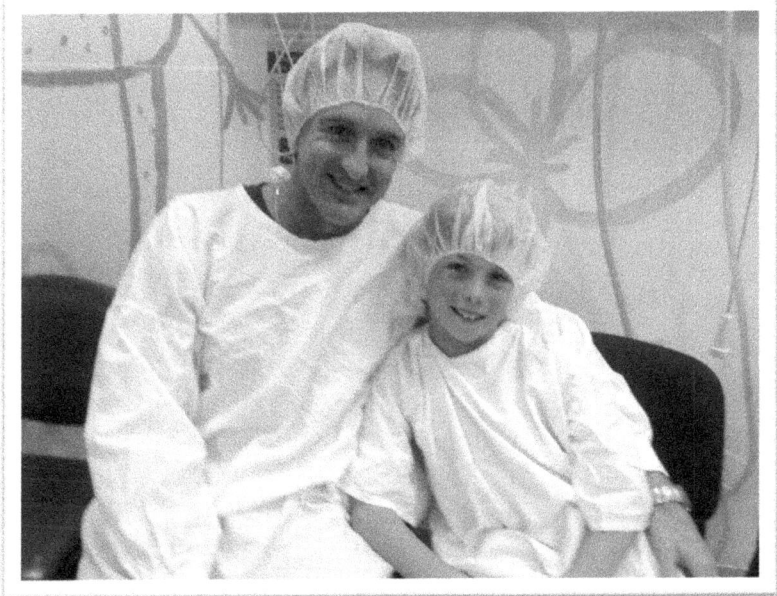
Dad and me before my portacath insertion surgery.

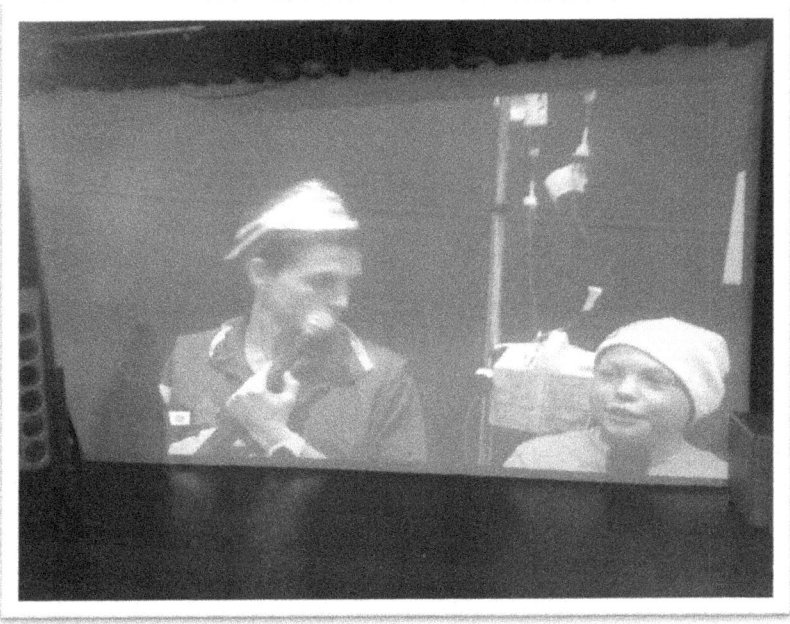
The infamous shark quiz with Captain Starlight.

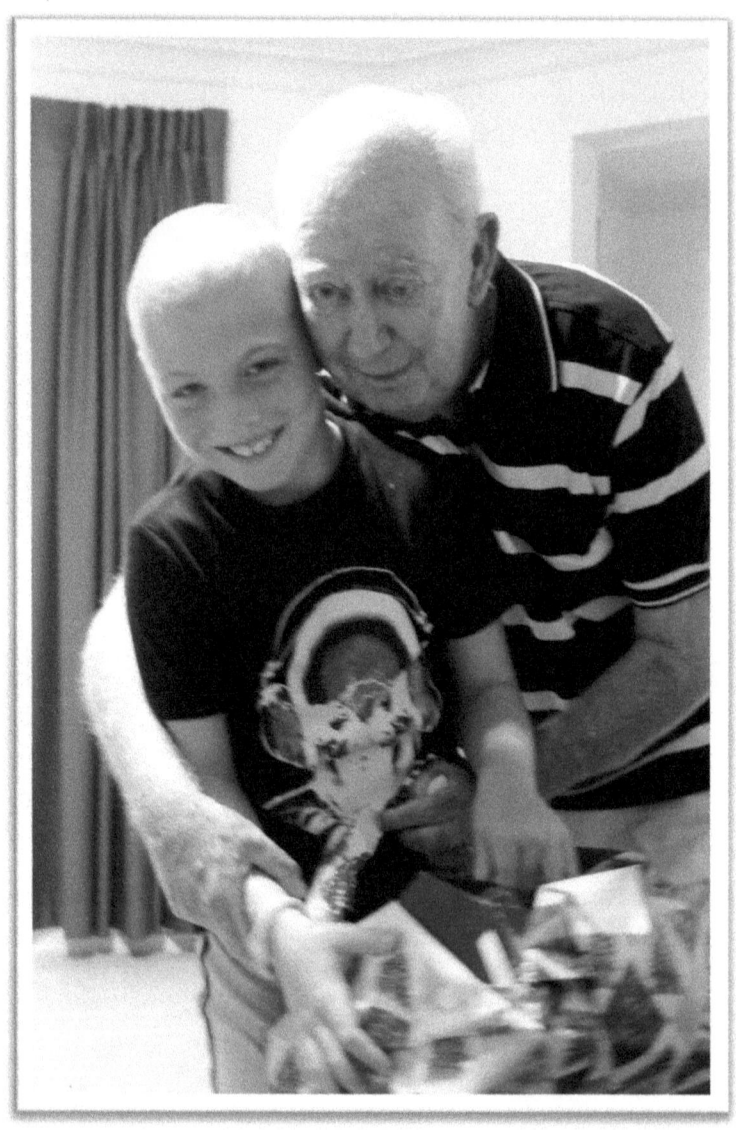

My late grandfather Bazza and me on Christmas Day.

Angus Cunningham

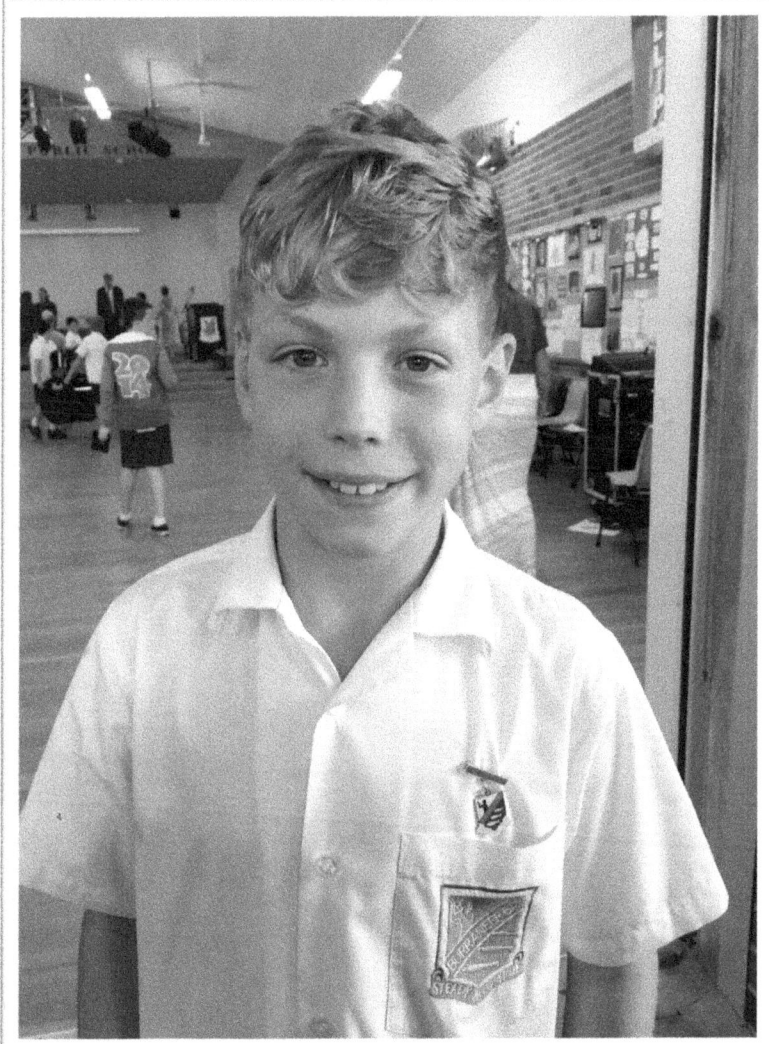

First photo as school captain, 2014.

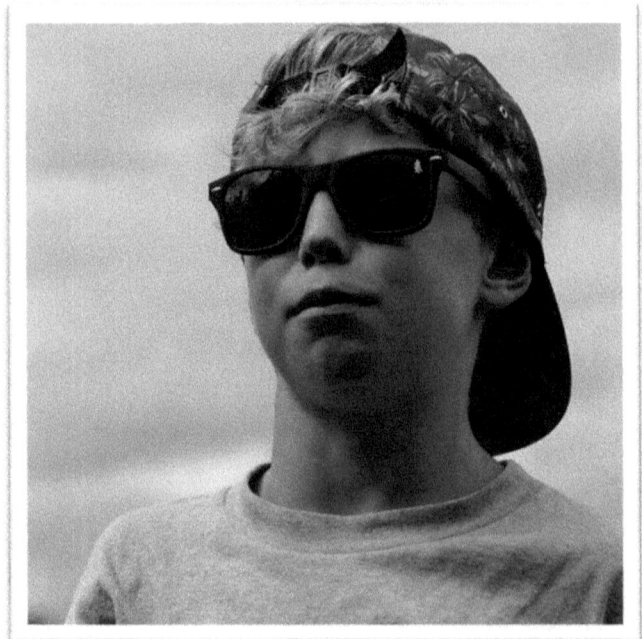

Narooma, January 2015.

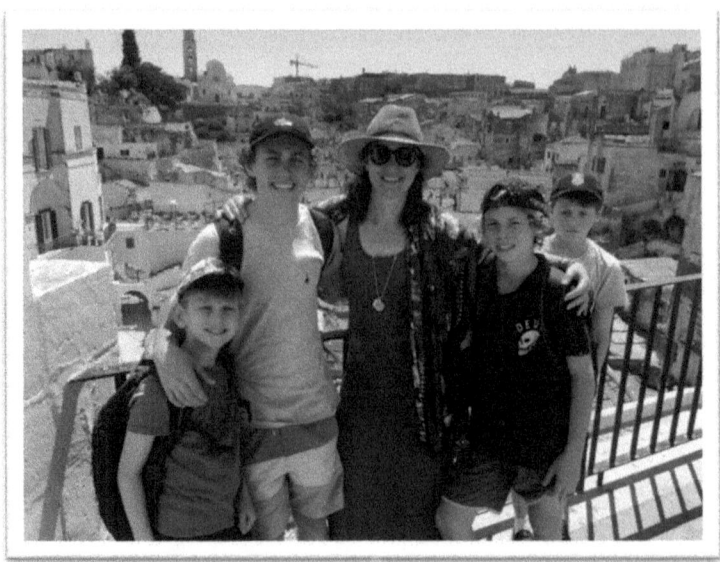

Family trip with Mum, Henry, Noah, Darcy, and me.

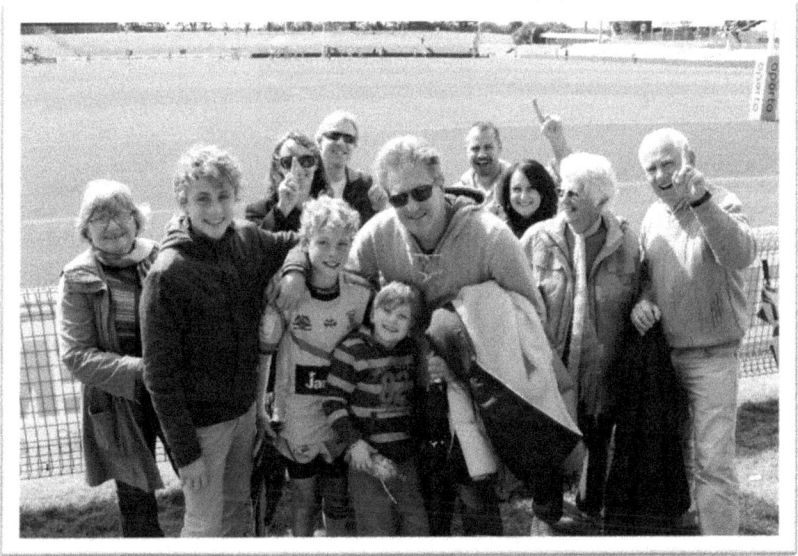
Grand final win with my family. Up De La!

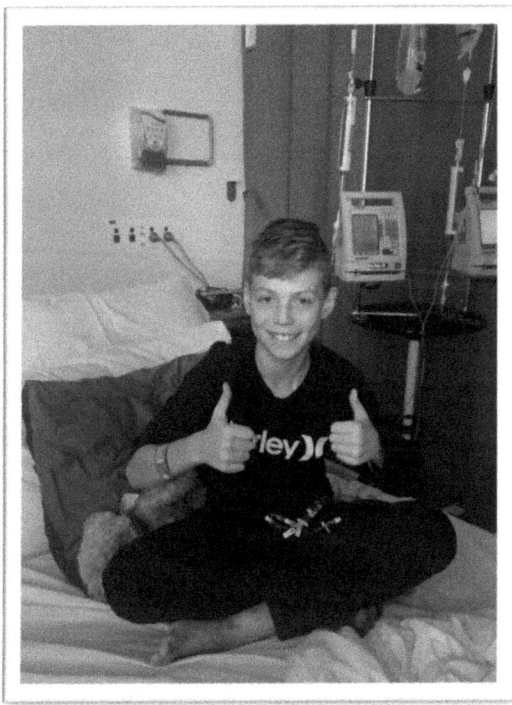
Cancer recurrence in 2015, trying to keep the hair.

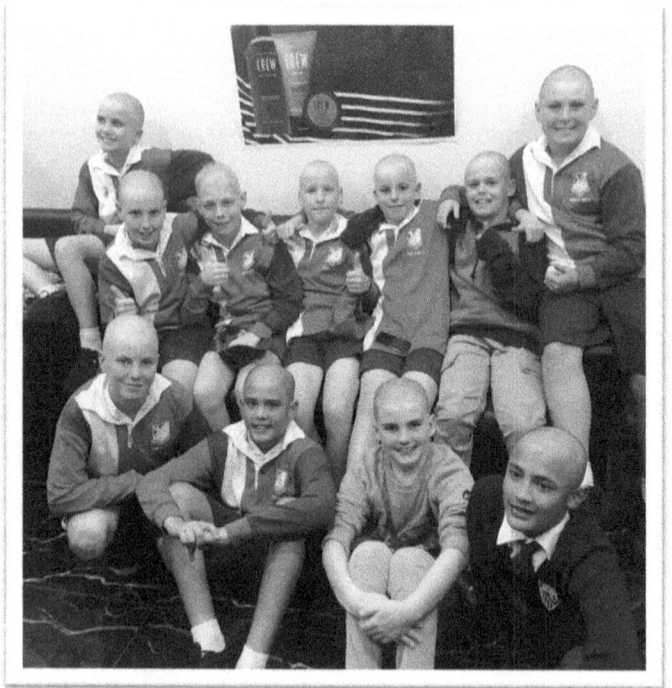

2015, I had the best mates in the world. Round two hair shave.

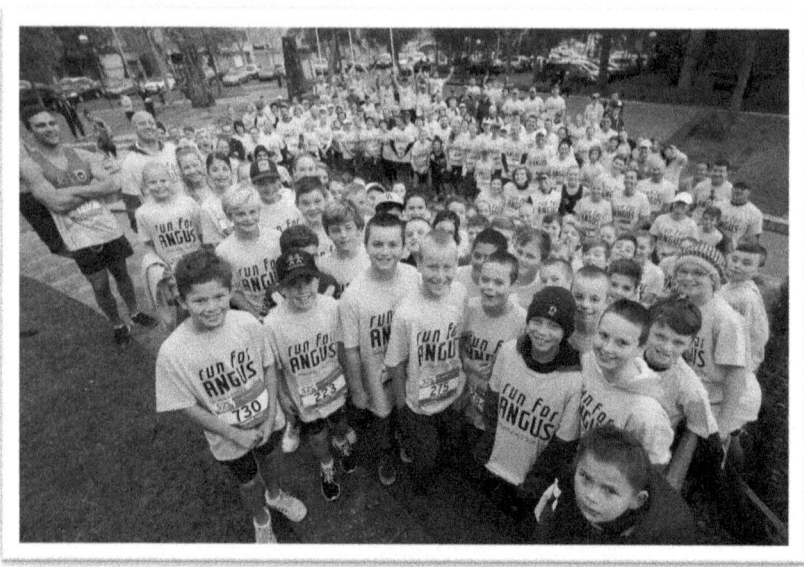

Run 4 Angus, organised by Aaron Raper. Just one of the many things the Shire community did to support my family and me.

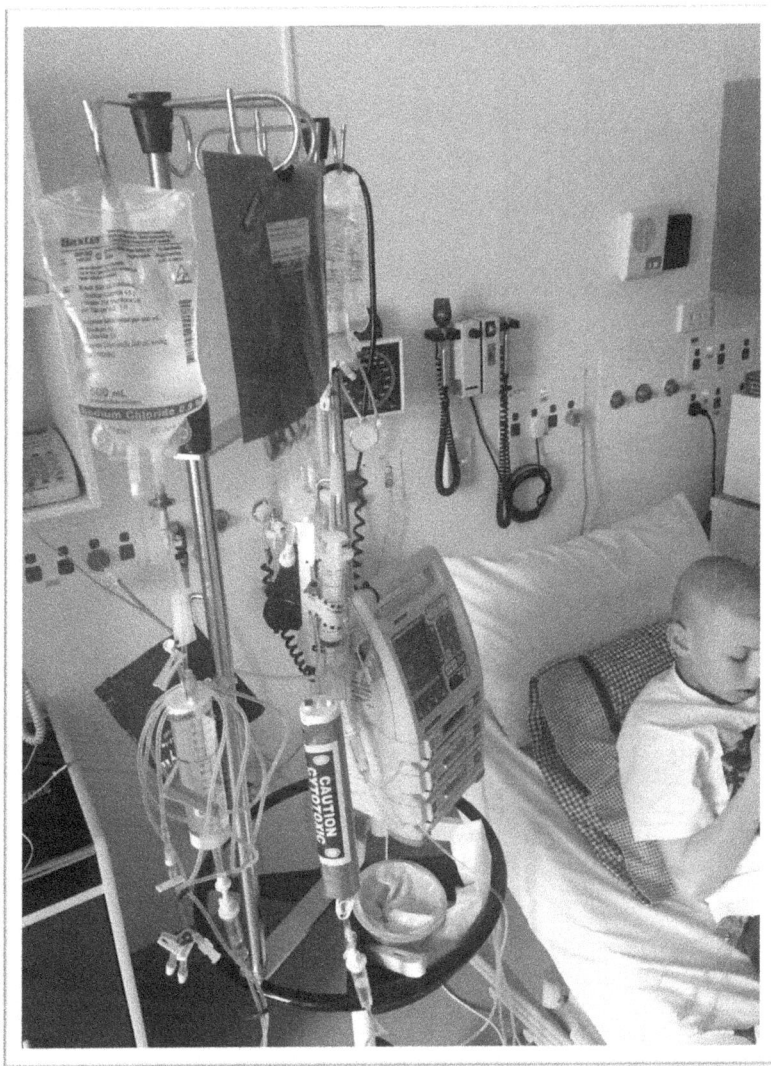

ICE chemotherapy protocol. Looks like more pump than boy!

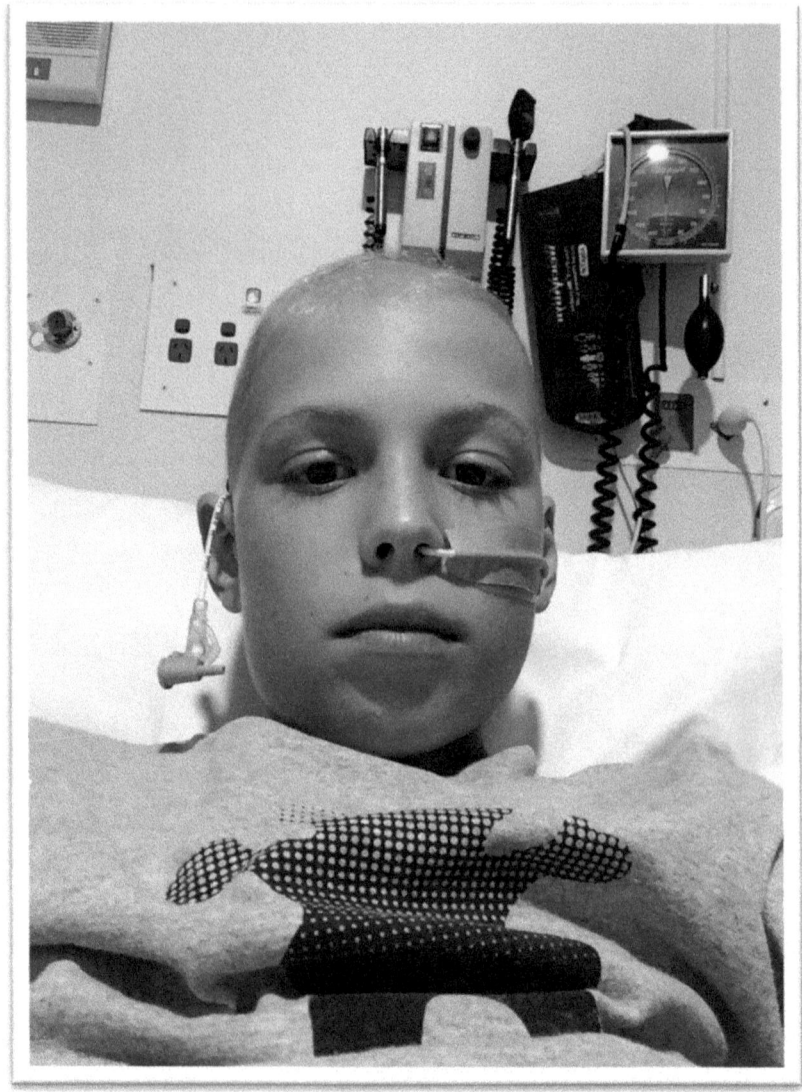

Feeding tube after it had been put in.

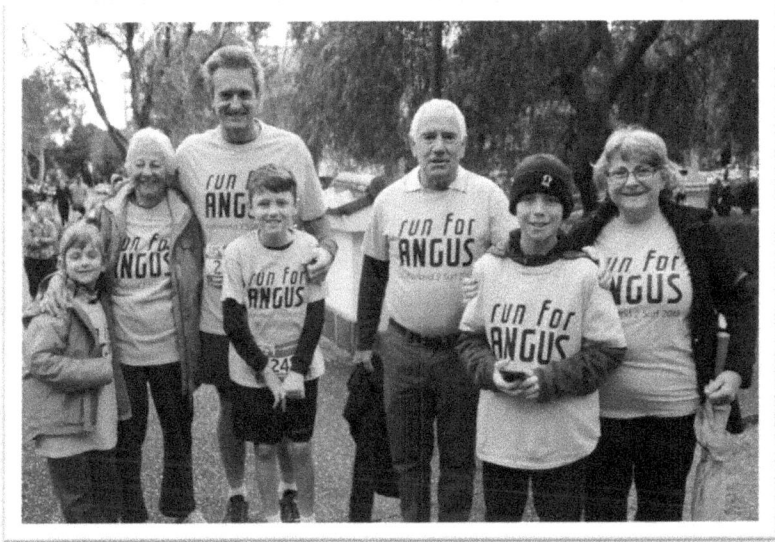

Another great photo with my grandparents, Nanna, Dad, and my brothers Noah, Darcy, and me. All rocking the beautiful blue Run 4 Angus shirt.

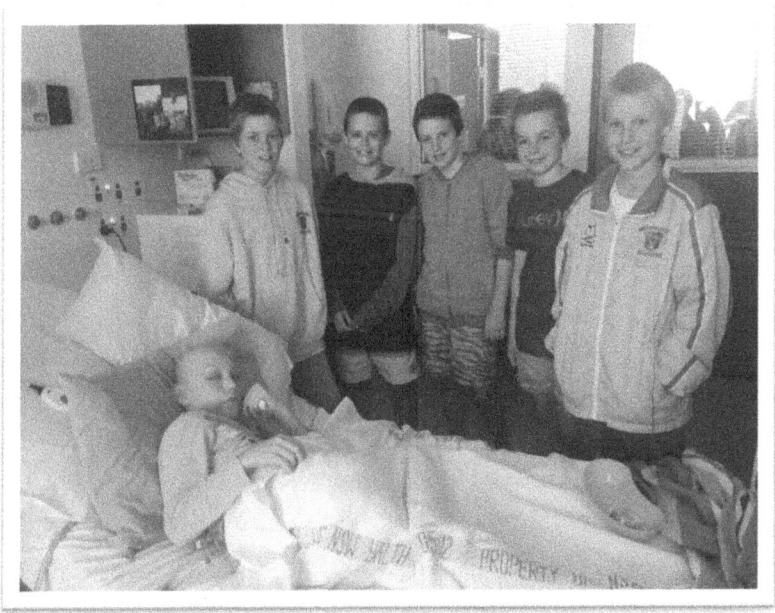

Surprise visit from my best mates, from left to right: Reid, Lachy, Jarvis, Vaughan, and Kai. Many tears were shed that day, thank you boys!

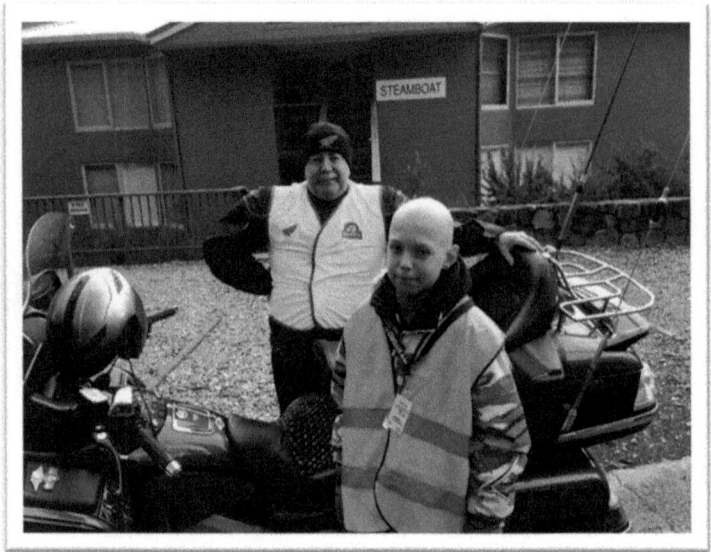

A nice memory from the Snowy Ride in 2014 that I looked at during my isolation period.

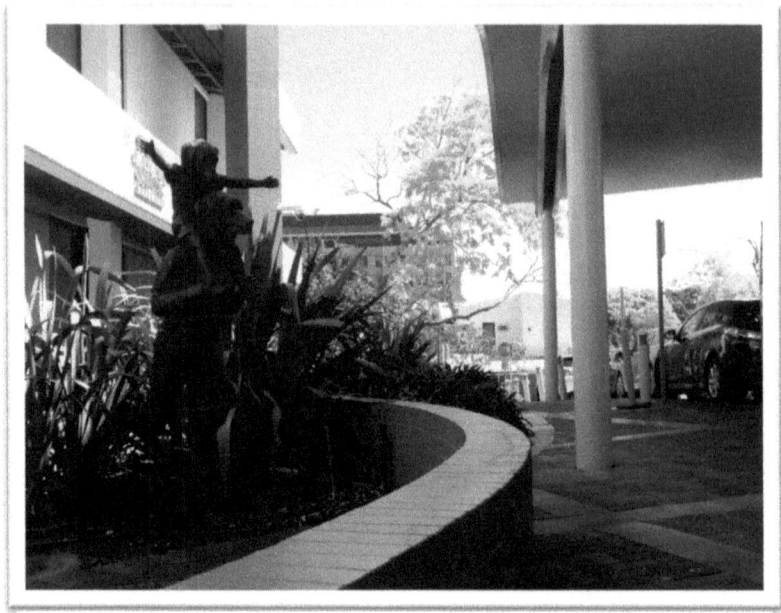

My first glimpse of the outside world after my autologous stem cell transplant. This simple photo represents so much.

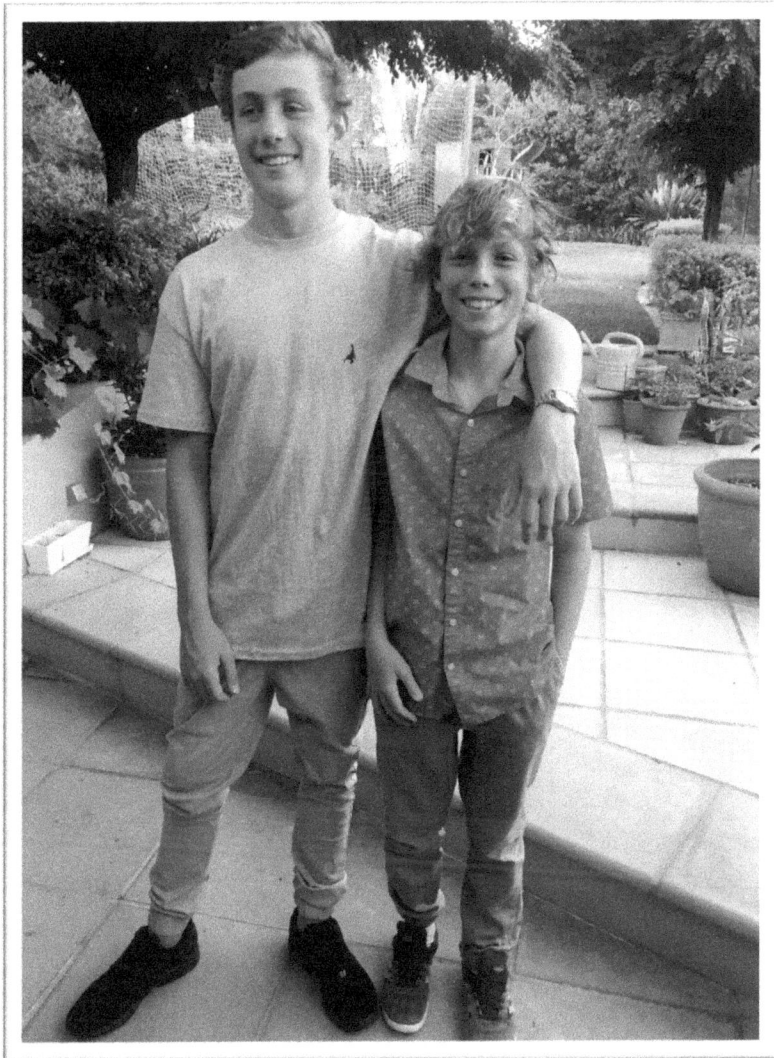

I let the hair grow out. Henry and me at Henry's 16th birthday.

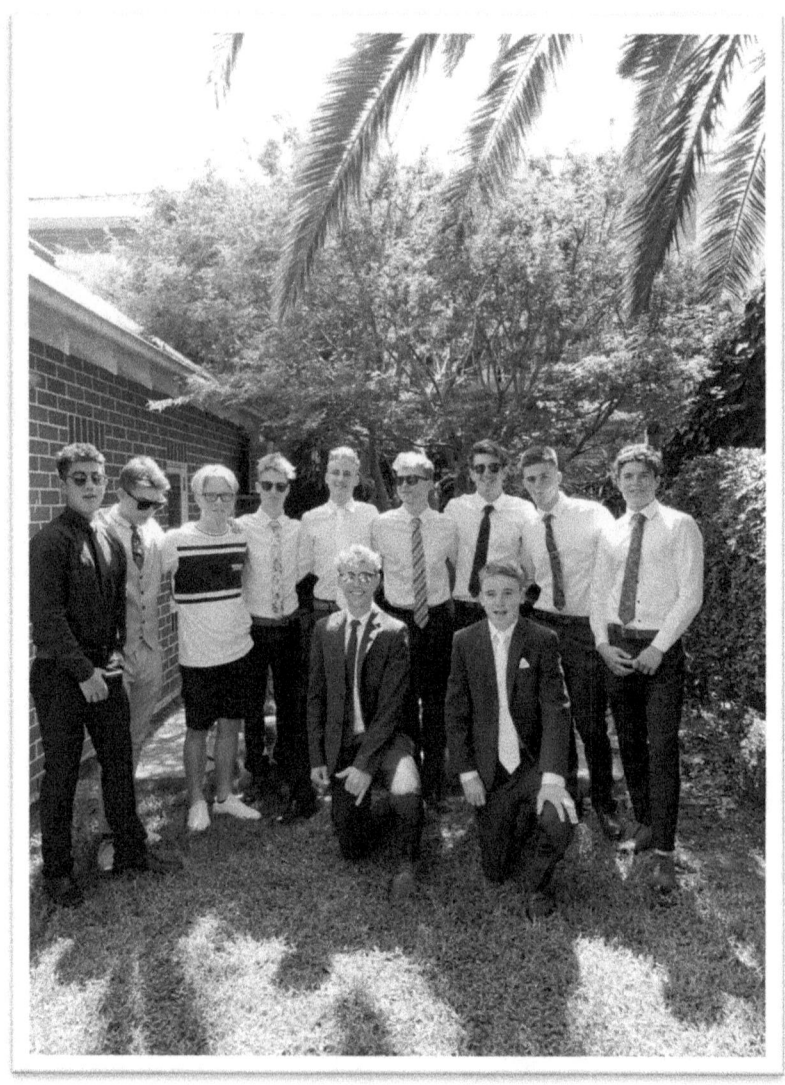
My mates and me before our Year 10 formal.

Angus Cunningham

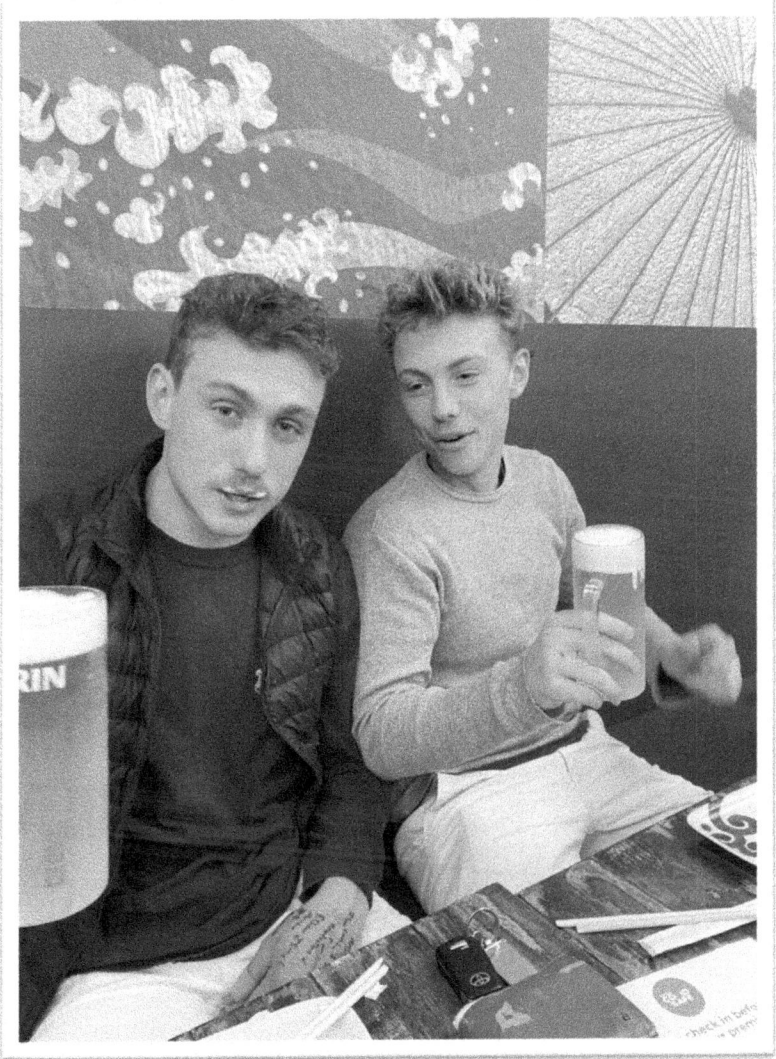

First legal beer when I was 18 with my brother Henry.

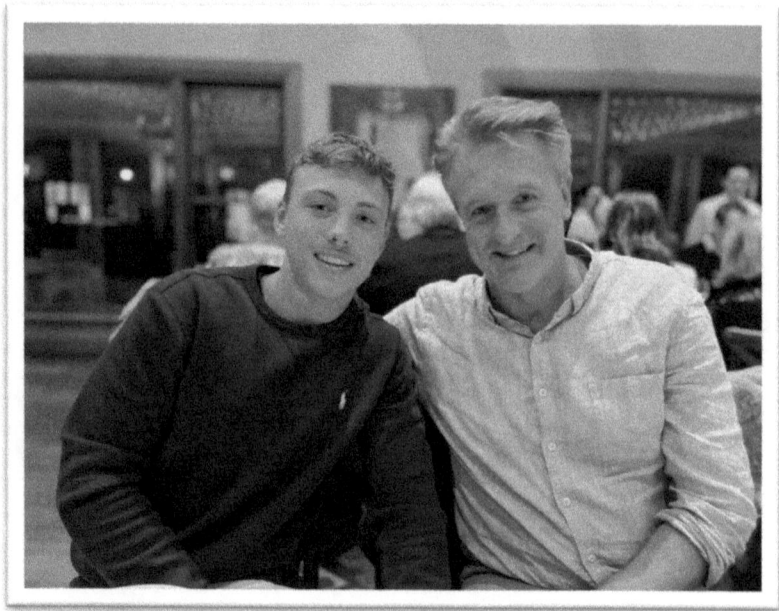

Dad and me at the 10-year Rare Cancers anniversary dinner.

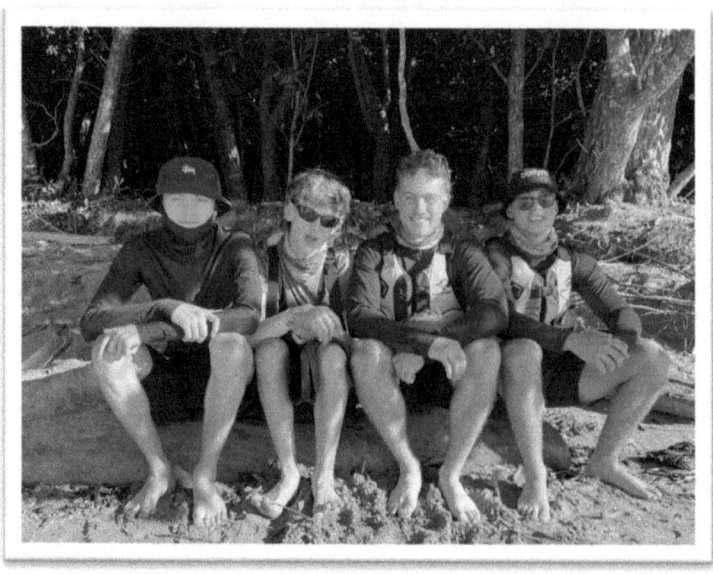

HAND taking on Hinchinbrook Island.

Angus Cunningham

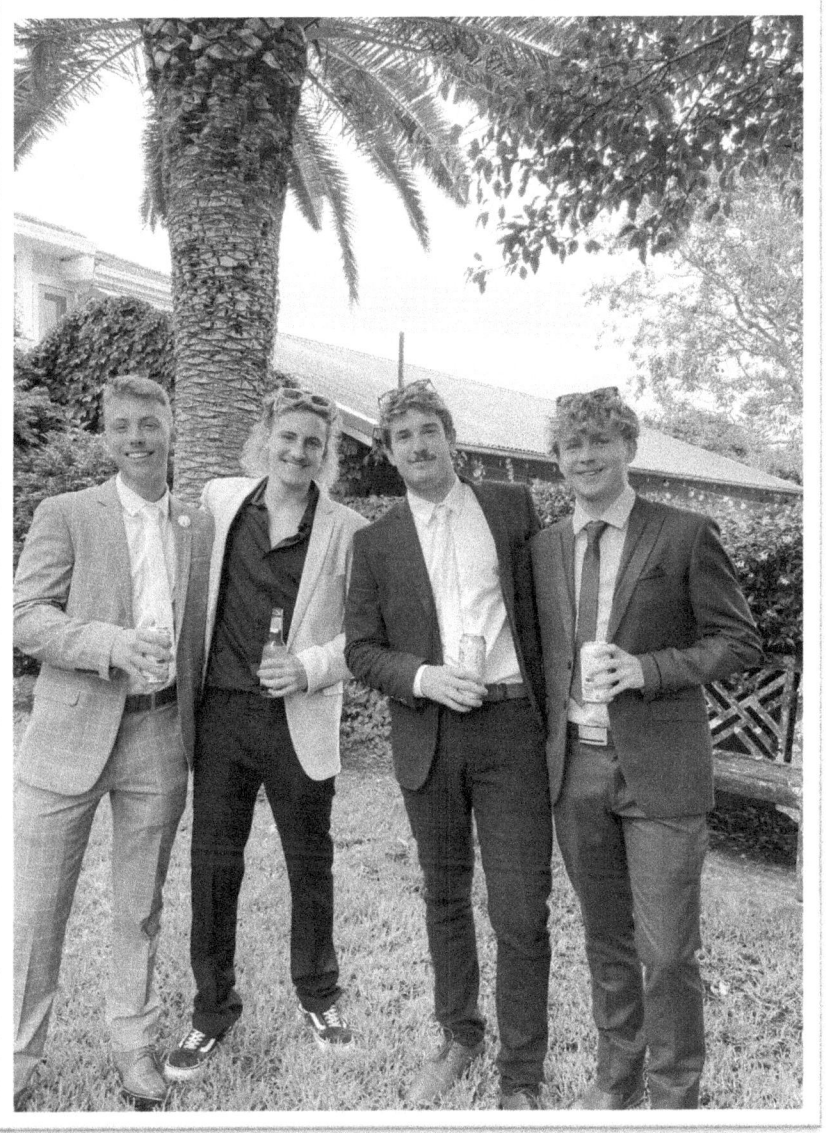

Year 12 formal photo with my mates. I'm on the left, next to Zayne, Guy, and Kailan.

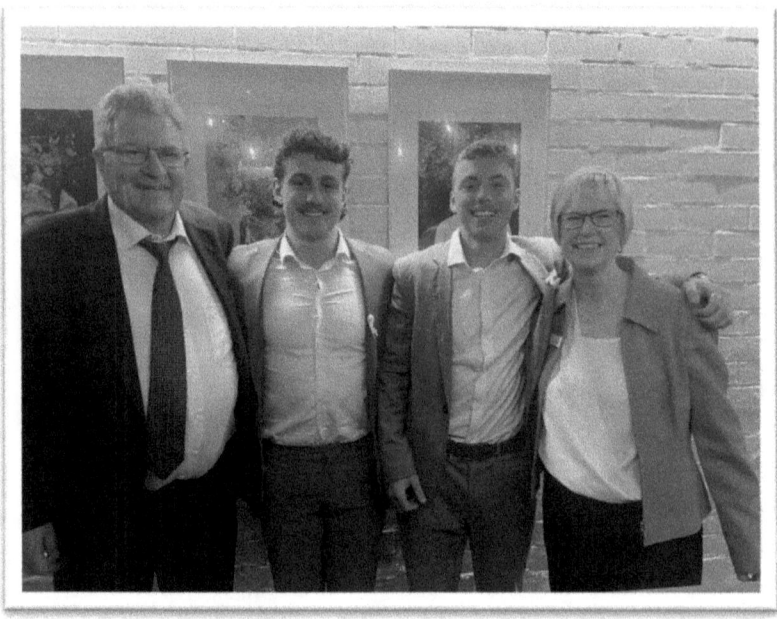

Henry and me with Richard and Kate Vines after my Parliament House speech for CanForum 2022.

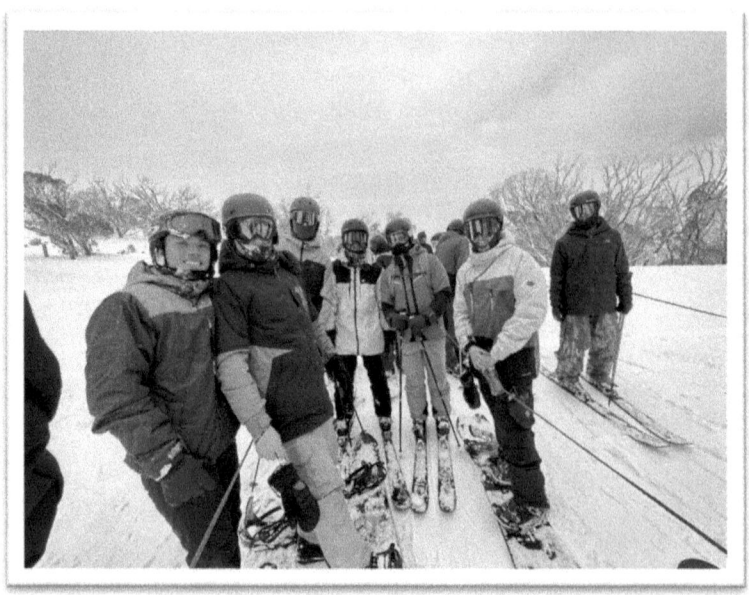

My mates and me at the snow in 2023. What a fantastic few days!

Angus Cunningham

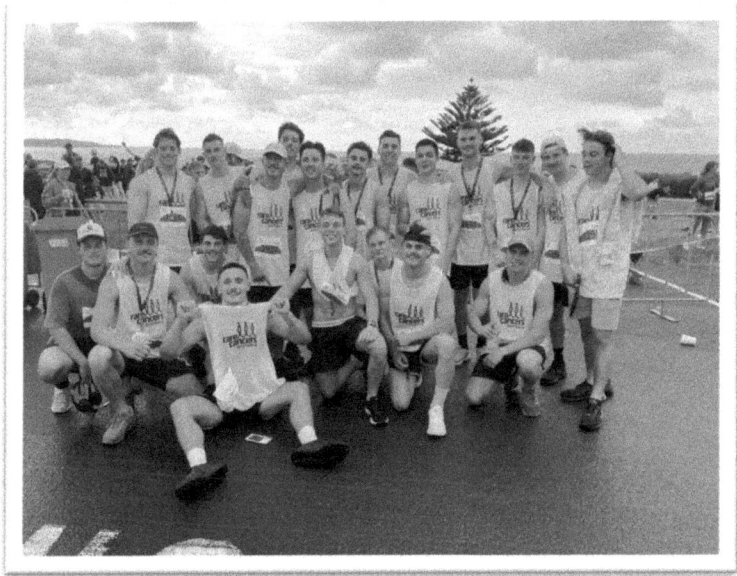

Rare Cancers fundraiser that Lachy Woodger and I set up, with a few of the boys who ran it with us. Great effort lads!

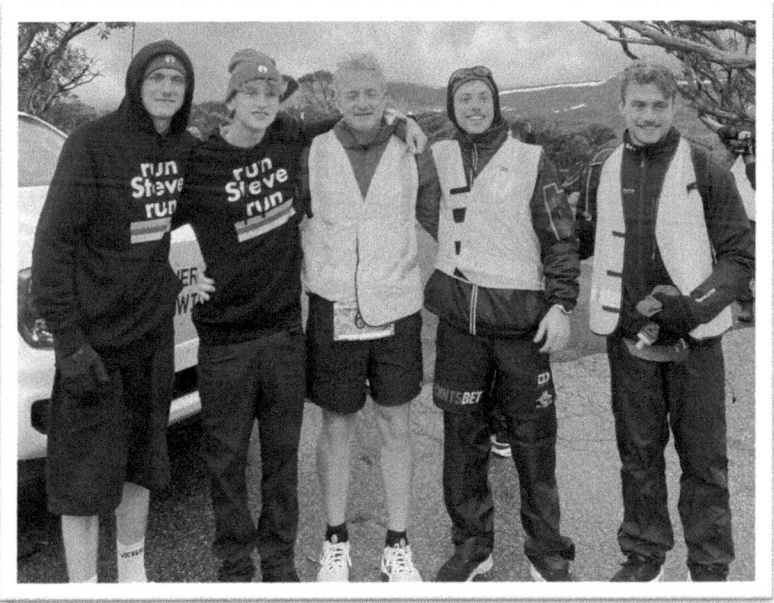

My family with Dad after his Coast2Kosci run of 240 km.

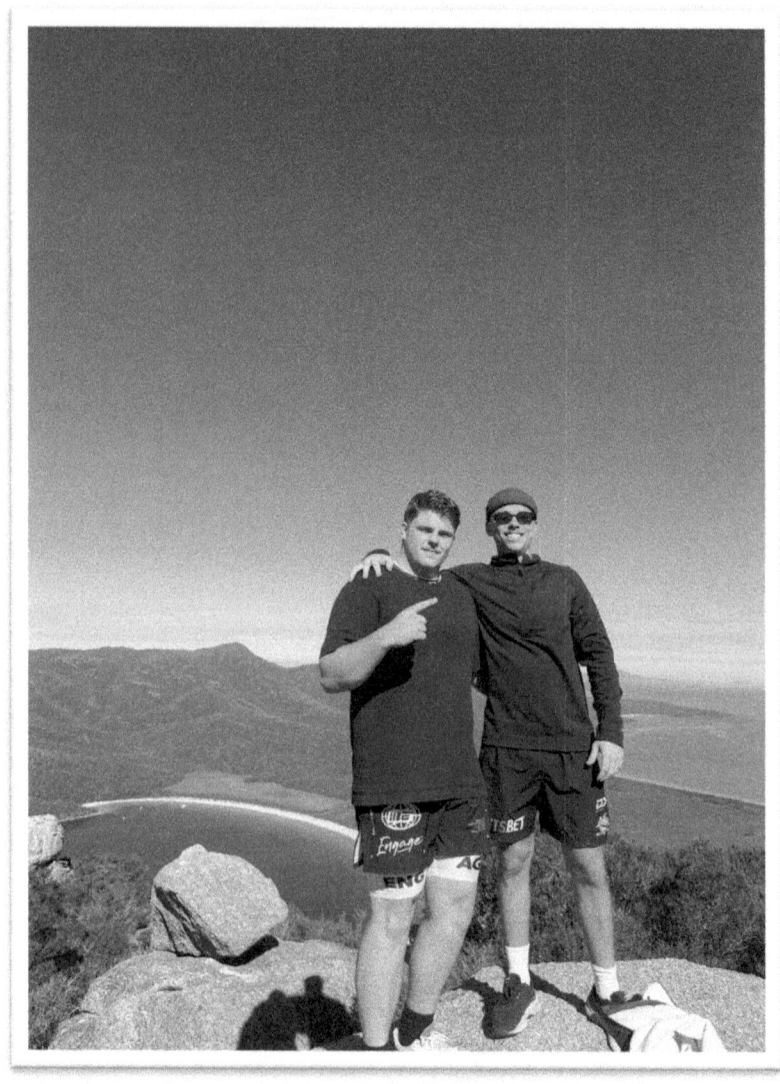

My good mate Kody and me celebrating my 21st birthday climbing a mountain in Tasmania.

Angus Cunningham

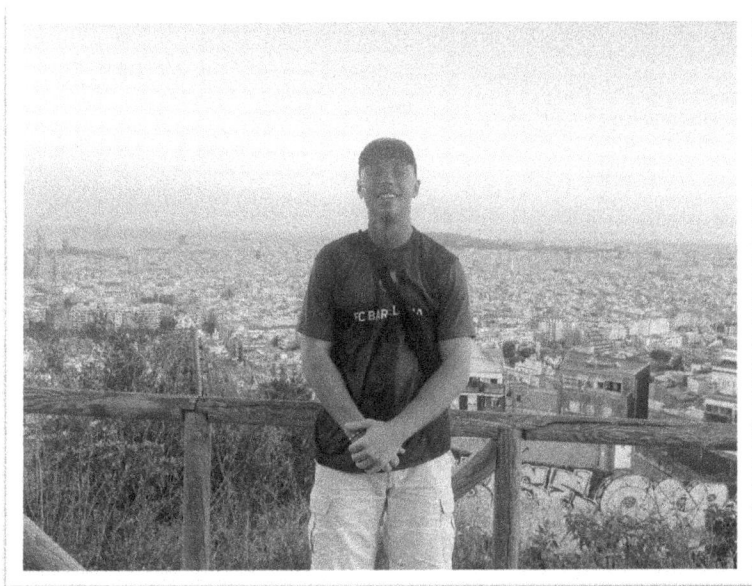

Solo travelling in Barcelona for university. What a great experience meeting many new friends across the world and trying to navigate that beautiful city.

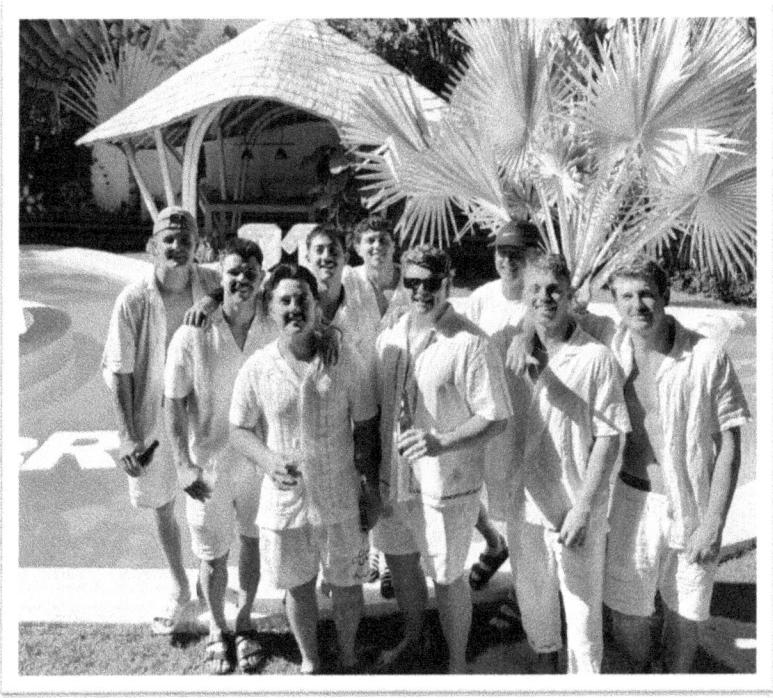

Kody's 21st birthday in Bali with all my mates.

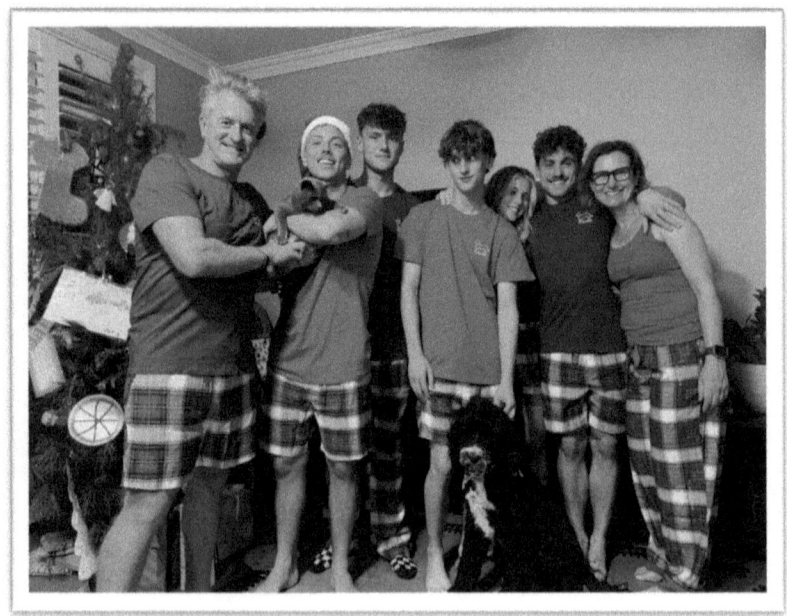

Cunningham family Christmas photo in matching PJs.

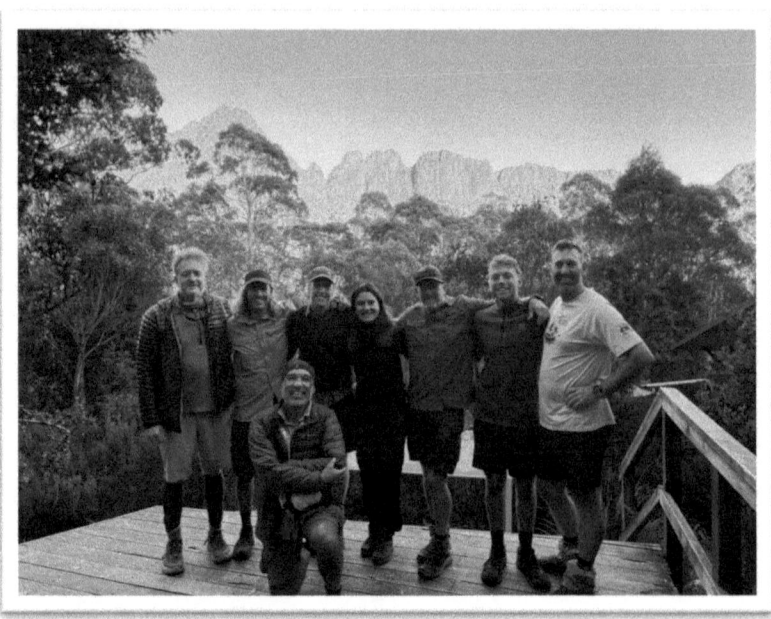

The hiking crew that hiked the Overland Track trail. One of the best weeks of my life!

Acknowledgements

Being sick with childhood cancer was the worst, and the hardest thing was knowing I couldn't avoid it. Even when I tried everything, it still came for me. However, what made a huge difference was the support that I received from the people around me. My Sutherland Shire community rallied around my family and me, and I'll never forget how supported and blessed we felt throughout the journey. Grandma and Pop, Bazza and Nanna, and my uncles, cousins and aunties – thank you so much for being there for us. It was a difficult time, but with everyone's help, it made a huge difference. Special shout out to Burraneer Bay PS, De La Salle JRLFC, and also both Cronulla Seagulls Cricket and Soccer clubs for the help.

Another massive shoutout to everyone that helped my family and me through these difficult times. All the amazing people that dropped my brothers to school or made them dinner whilst I was in the hospital. It is impossible to mention everyone, but it was enormously appreciated, and I hope you know that it is not forgotten what you guys did. Aunty Steph, buying me boxes of fantastic crackers to keep me eating when it felt impossible.

Thanks to Aaron Raper for allowing me to meet the Cronulla Sharks NRL team and getting me in touch with the club. They were and still are my favourite team; it was such a cool experience. All the players treated me like family, with Todd Carney even giving me his boots, which I still have to this day. I remember Andrew Fifita even FaceTiming me once; it was awesome. The things the Cronulla Sharks did for me – behind closed doors and with no media presence or anything – just show what the club does for the community, and they are things I will never forget. I wish I had kept in contact with the club, but after my first diagnosis, I really tried to forget about everything and move on. But this is just the start, and I want my gratitude for all the lovely people who helped me to be a constant reminder of how their kindness and support shaped every step of this journey.

My school teachers throughout my education journey, thank you for your support.

Dr Toby Trahair, you are an amazing human, and you work doesn't go unnoticed. My family and I will never be able to thank you enough for what you did! No matter what time of the day you were happy to talk to Mum and Dad, and offer us support. We will never forget that.

To my friends, past and present, you guys have had my back through thick and thin and I will always appreciate every single one of you. There are way too many to mention, but you know who you are.

A heartfelt thank you to Dr Juliette Lachemeier, managing editor of The Erudite Pen, who helped bring this story to life.

Lastly, Kate and Richard Vines and Rare Cancers Australia, your charity is amazing, and it gives people like me another chance. The unwavering support you had for me and my family was second to none, and I hope you guys enjoy the book.

ABOUT THE AUTHOR

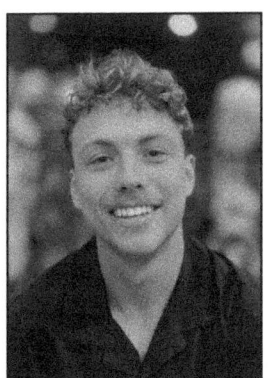

Angus Cunningham is a survivor, storyteller and passionate advocate for children and families affected by cancer. Twice before the age of twelve he faced childhood cancer, an experience that shaped not only his resilience but also his outlook on life.

Now twenty-two, Angus shares his journey in *Twice Before Twelve: A Journey Through Childhood Cancer*, a memoir that is raw, funny, wise and filled with gratitude. His story honours the love of family, the loyalty of friends and the generosity of a community that walked beside him through the darkest of times.

Beyond writing, Angus is an active supporter of Rare Cancers Australia, raising funds and awareness for those still fighting. He has spoken at Parliament House for CanForum (2022) and first appeared on *A Current Affair* in 2015, inspiring many with his courage and optimism.

A proud fan of the NRL Cronulla Sharks, Angus continues to champion hope, kindness and resilience, reminding others that even in life's toughest battles, light can always be found.

Enjoyed the book? You can follow the author at:

Facebook: Angus Cunningham

Instagram: Angus.Cunningham Author

LinkedIn: Angus Cunningham

If you liked the book, please leave a review on Amazon, Goodreads or with the author directly. Reviews are invaluable in supporting an author's hard work and are greatly appreciated.

www.ingramcontent.com/pod-product-compliance
Lightning Source LLC
LaVergne TN
LVHW051218070526
838200LV00064B/4954